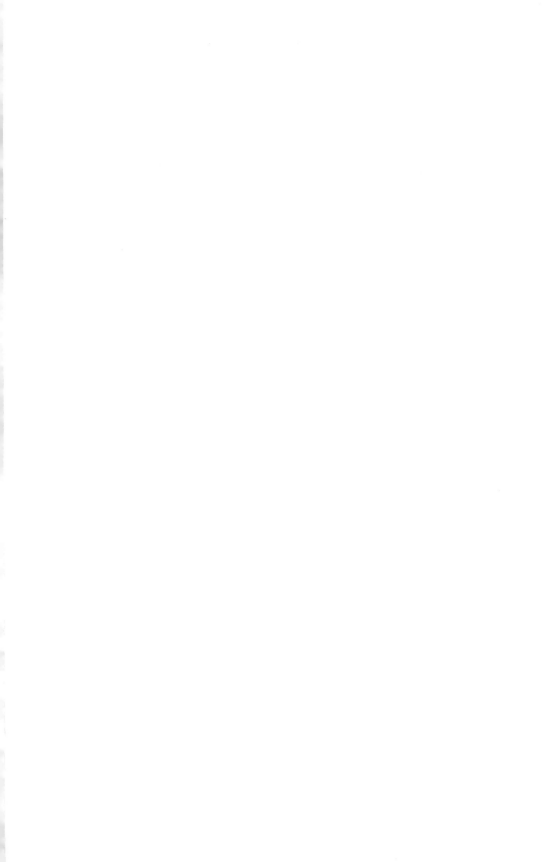

Go Lavishly Natural

100+ Recipes
for Healthy Natural Hair, Mind, & Soul

Erica K. King, PhD

BALBOA.
PRESS

A DIVISION OF HAY HOUSE

Balboa Press books may be ordered through booksellers or by contacting:

Balboa Press
A Division of Hay House
1663 Liberty Drive
Bloomington, IN 47403
www.balboapress.com
1 (877) 407-4847

Because of the dynamic nature of the Internet, any web addresses or links contained in this book may have changed since publication and may no longer be valid. The views expressed in this work are solely those of the author and do not necessarily reflect the views of the publisher, and the publisher hereby disclaims any responsibility for them.

The author of this book does not dispense medical advice or prescribe the use of any technique as a form of treatment for physical, emotional, or medical problems without the advice of a physician, either directly or indirectly. The intent of the author is only to offer information of a general nature to help you in your quest for emotional and spiritual well-being. In the event you use any of the information in this book for yourself, which is your constitutional right, the author and the publisher assume no responsibility for your actions.

Any people depicted in stock imagery provided by Thinkstock are models, and such images are being used for illustrative purposes only.
Certain stock imagery © Thinkstock.

Print information available on the last page.

ISBN: 978-1-5043-7873-4 (sc)
ISBN: 978-1-5043-7874-1 (hc)
ISBN: 978-1-5043-7875-8 (e)

Library of Congress Control Number: 2017906519

Balboa Press rev. date: 08/18/2017

To Asia, Laila, and Damon (DJ), I love you.

CONTENTS

INTRODUCTION

Most people don't have a visceral reaction to honey like I do. Not that honey that comes in the cute bear container. I'm talking about the sheer ecstasy of fresh, raw, organic honey.

Just opening a jar is a ritual for me.

I use honey for everything: my relaxing baths, just about every hair product I make, skin cleansers, conditioners, and moisturizers. I almost cried when I bought my first jar of local, raw honey from a bee farmer (he sells it sometimes on the corner of 99th & Thomas). It was like buying liquid gold!

When my husband brings me this, or big bouquets of lacinato kale, it's better than roses ... and there are few things better than roses—maybe tulips, hydrangea, and birds of paradise, but I digress.

I wasn't always a weeping naturalista blogging and vlogging about honey and all-things-natural hair. I started making my own products because I had to. I could handle my own skin changes and challenges, but watching my kids' discomfort, particularly due to allergies, was overwhelming.

A few of the allergies in our home include: *milk, dairy (casein), shellfish, treenuts, peanuts, soy, fish, and gluten.* I won't even talk about the food sensitivities.

Why Do I Tell You This?

Since you're reading *Go Lavishly Natural*, I know you're serious about your health. You're looking for natural, maybe even organic recipes that are easy to follow but also fulfill a need.

Perhaps you live with allergies like my family and seek natural, allergy-free alternatives. Maybe you're interested in healthier hair and the best foods for hair retention. Or perhaps you're one of the millions who have experienced hair thinning, hair breakage, or hair loss and want natural solutions.

Finding homemade remedies that work for thick, luscious, kinky, curly hair may have become part of your natural hair journey. That's what I'm here for—*to provide you great recipes that make your life easier and help you fulfill your naturalista goals!*

There are over a hundred recipes in these pages to help you fully stock your healthy home salon: do-it-yourself (DIY) hair products, body-care goodies, healing foods, fresh green drinks, and a 21-day relaxation diet.

Naturalistas definitely want to know what's in their hair products, and these discoveries often highlight other lifestyle areas they'd like to change. Being natural goes beyond hair care and may include:

- ✓ *investing in more organic, natural products*
- ✓ *eating a more natural, plant-based based diet*
- ✓ *using complementary and integrative health practices for healing and prevention*
- ✓ *making your own natural hair and body-care products*

Go Lavishly Natural shares recipes I've created through the years for myself, family, clients, and friends. Most of them I share on my blog, LavishlyNatutural.com—DIY Recipes for 4C Natural Hair, Health and Wellness.

The recipes in this book have helped me grow my hair back after hair breakage, thinning, and alopecia. They've contributed to helping me and my family heal numerous conditions, including food sensitivities, eczema, fibroids, obesity, and high blood pressure. They're even helping my son recover from the debilitating effects of autism.

Amen & Hallelujah!

May all the recipes in this book serve you well. They have been a joy to make and to share. May they bring you as much joy and healing as they have brought me, my family, and the Lavishly Natural Community.

Abundant Love & Raw Honey,
Erica

Chapter 1

Natural Hair and Body Care: DIY Basics for the Modern Naturalista

You are the sum total of everything you've ever seen, heard, eaten, smelled, been told, forgot—it's all there. … Everything influences each of us, and because of that I try to make sure that my experiences are positive.
Maya Angelou

Before we get started, I'd like to get a few things off my hair. First, what is a modern naturalista, and Is being a naturalista just related to hair?

I define a naturalista in three ways:

1. *Someone who doesn't chemically relax his or her hair*
2. *Someone who has a natural approach to or philosophy of health, life, mind, body, and food*
3. *Someone who has a natural approach to healing, specifically with medical and mental conditions*

You may find that you're all three, one more than the others, or none at all. Perhaps you're more of a naturalist. The word naturalista comes from the French word *naturaliste*. Its definitions include:

- **A person who studies nature, especially by direct observation of animals and plants**
- **A person who believes in or practices naturalism in any form**

As someone who is reading this book, you are an official naturalista! I know you have an interest in the best ingredients and the highest-quality products that work best for your hair and skin. You don't have to wear your hair naturally to enjoy that—but if you do, the recipes in this book will complement your current regime and may eventually become all you need to care for your gorgeous natural hair!

How To Use This Book

You can read this book straight through, or pick and choose your favorite recipes and chapters. It was written so that you could turn to a page and find something that works for you! You can also skip right to The Relaxation Diet (pg.) at any time. Each day is a complete act of relaxation:)

Getting Started | How to Make Your Own Natural Hair Care Line

Start with the Products You'd Like to Make

Do you love hair butters?

Are luscious, thick conditioners your thing?

When my hair fell out (again) in 2011, I needed everything—a new shampoo, an oil-free conditioner, leave-ins, and anything that offered moisture.

I suggest picking two to three products you'd really like to make (try a mega hair-growth serum, page 56, or coconut shea butter, page 60) and go from there. Don't concern yourself with how easy or hard it will be to make, or what ingredients are required.

Once you have your products, move on to step 2: identifying the right ingredients for your hair.

Identifying What Works

Now that you know what you want to make, it's time to identify the ingredients you'll be working with for your own luscious creations. To do this, we'll need to look at your favorite hair products. I'll show you how to create your own list when we make our *Mega Hair-Growth Oil* in Chapter 10.

Quick Tip

You'll want to include the ingredients, even if they aren't natural. Why? This product is working for your hair, so before you remove anything, we'll see if there are any natural alternatives for that ingredient.

Check Your Ingredients—On Everything

The next time you're ready to buy or use your favorite products, check your ingredients. I love almond oil, walnut oil, and macadamia oil, which are all found in many natural products—but with the severe nut allergies in my family, they're out, out, and out. I also don't want toxic parabens in my shampoos or conditioners.

Parabens are often used as preservatives in foods, pharmaceuticals, and cosmetics. They keep funkiness from growing in your hair products with their antifungal and antibacterial properties. The FDA lists methylparaben, propylparaben, butylparaben, and ethylparaben as the most common parabens found in our products. Although parabens may provide some benefits to our cosmetic formulations, they also come with some baggage.

Paraben Exposé *(Watch Out For These In Your Products)*

Methylparabens are often listed as 4-hydroxy-methyl ester benzoic acid, and sodium salt in your ingredients. Methylparabens and each of the parabens that follow, mimic estrogen and can disrupt the endocrine system.[25,]

Propylparabens are often used as fragrance. This paraben can cause endocrine (hormone) disruptions that include birth defects, developmental delays, and cancerous tumors.[26] Other names you might see proplyparabens listed as include, potassium salt propylparaben, propyl 4-hydroxybenzoate, and benzoic acid.

Butylparabens (also called benzoic acid, sodium salt, 4-hydroxy-butyl ester benzoic acid)[22] can cause skin irritation, disrupt the cellular structure and function of your organs, and weaken the immune system.

Last but not least, ethylparabens are often used as a preservative and a fragrance. Ethylparabens have been linked to—you guessed it—disrupting the hormones and cycles of the body[20, 24] (menstrual cycles, hair growth cycles, etc.). The good news is that of all the parabens, it seems to rate the lowest on the toxicity scale. Yay!

What's That In Your Conditioner?

Have you ever heard another naturalista say she hates *cones* and had no idea what she was talking about? More than likely, it was little d, dimethicone.

Dimethicone is a silicone-based polymer[53] (part of the rubber family; plastic) that works as a conditioning emollient. It's a common ingredient in most conditioners. It provides slip and lubrication to hair and skin products and reduces greasiness in creams and oils. It's often the ingredient that makes your conditioner so easy to wash out.

When used over time, dimethicone can cause product buildup on your hair, seal off your hair cuticles' ability to absorb moisture, and weigh your hair down. EWG lists dimethicone as a *moderate health concern* because it's been linked to non-reproductive organ system toxicity.

Make Your First DIY Recipe

We've covered how to get started making your hair care line, which ingredients to use, and which ones to keep out of your natural goodies. Let's get this party started with the very first products we use to keep our hair fresh and clean! In the next section, we'll cover the best homemade shampoos that clean your hair and nourish your spirit.

Chapter 2

Take the Challenge

If you don't understand yourself you don't understand anybody else.
—Nikki Giovanni

In 2013 while lying on the Keawakapu Beach in Maui, I had two revelations. One, never forget sunscreen again, and two, I should start a hair challenge. Something had to change with Lavishly Natural. We were living in Maui at the time, and I didn't have the same access to hair and body care ingredients like I had in Arizona. Shipping was expensive, and what I was able to bring was limited. I learned how to do everything with clay, vanilla oil, coconut oil, and shea butter! It was a challenge with three luscious heads of natural hair to do every day.

I had a total of 1,100 e-mail subscribers and an idea that each week for ninety days (the standard time of most wonderful hair challenges), I would share a tip we could use to grow and care for our healthy hair. That first year, it was me and one other naturalista. Success! From that moment on, every winter, I ran the challenge, and it got bigger and bigger. It's now been shared over 50,000 times and counting!

Lavishly Natural's Healthy Hair Challenge

Thousands of women and young girls have participated in the challenge, and I invite you to join now too! Simply go to EricaKKing.com/lavishlynatural and sign up for the automated thirty-day course. I'll come to your inbox every day and challenge you to complete one exercise a day. The activities don't take long to complete, and you may recognize some of the recipes in this book.

You're going to love it, and I'm not the least bit biased.

Are You Part of the Lavishly Natural Goddess Community?

If you have read this book and still have not signed up for my Lavishly Natural Updates, stop right now and take your beautiful self here: LavishlyNatural.com. There, you can sign up for my weekly newsletter and get information about live courses and events! I share exclusive recipes and tips with my readers that you cannot find anywhere else, so come, and bring your hair.

Relax Goddess

In the last part of this book, you will find the Twenty-One-Day Relaxation Diet. It's a fun way to incorporate many of the recipes in this book into a simple daily practice. It will also help reduce your current stress level and bring peace to your mind and body.

After the Twenty-One-Day Relaxation Diet, I've also included a shopping list (appendix B) that has all of the ingredients used in this book. You do not have to buy everything at once. You probably have most of the ingredients in your pantry already. At the end of the list, I share places where you can find natural, organic ingredients online. I shop from each of them for anything I can't buy locally. As always, look around and do your own research on everything that touches your hair and skin. Do not skip this step. You are your own expert, and your hair is fabulous!

Chapter 3

How to Make Your Own Shampoo

Most of the products for natural hair are rich, creamy, and completely indulgent—so much so that they can leave a little product buildup on the hair. This is normal, but if you have hard water, this little buildup can become a big problem.

The following recipes are wonderful for use any time you want to deeply cleanse and detoxify your hair. If you want a deeper detox, try the chelating cactus syrup. It's magical!

Six All-Natural Cleansers for Beautiful, Natural Hair

1. Soap Nut Foam Clarifying Shampoo
2. Erica's Bentonite Clay Wash
3. Chelating Cactus Syrup
4. Cherry Club Soda
5. Lavishly Natural's Herbal Shampoo
6. Super Bowl Clay Wash

#1 Soap Nut Foam Clarifying Shampoo

Looking for a foam based shampoo that won't leave product buildup?

Soap nut foam is the answer!

Soap nut cleansing has become a popular alternative to chemical detergents. Soap nuts, *(Sapindus mukorossi, also called soapberries),* contain an all-natural detergent called saponin. When the soap nut shell absorbs water, it releases saponin into the water. This fabulous foamy surfactant gently removes dirt, oils, and grime from your hair and clothes.

Ingredients

4 to 6 soap nuts
1 cup of water

Instructions

1. Add soap nuts to a small 2-quart pot.
2. Add water to the pot and bring soap nuts to a boil.
3. Reduce to low-medium heat. Let them simmer for 20 minutes.
4. Strain out the soap nuts. You can use these again by storing them in a plastic bag once they dry. Keep them in your refrigerator for up to 1 month.
5. Pour the liquid in a food processor or blender.
6. Blend or mix on high for 30 seconds. The soap nut wash should begin to foam up as you mix.
7. Place foam in a bottle with a pump or in a sealable jar.

How to Use Soap Nut Foam

Massage the foam into your hair and work it down your strands. Continue to massage your scalp gently with the shampoo. If you want a deeper cleanse, allow the shampoo to sit on your hair for up to 5 minutes. The foam will begin to disappear as you use it, but it's still cleaning.

Rinse and repeat if needed. Follow up with your favorite hair tea, conditioner, and styling aids.

Soap nut foam can be drying by itself, so make sure to condition after use.

#2 Erica's Bentonite Clay Wash

Bentonite clay is an ancient cleanser that originates from volcanic ash. When used as a cleanser, it pulls the dirt, oils, and buildup out of your hair. It deeply detangles coily, curly hair with ease.

Ingredients

3 tablespoons bentonite clay
3 tablespoons apple cider vinegar
2 tablespoons marshmallow root powder
1/2 cup aloe vera juice (add gradually)
2 tablespoons organic honey
1 tablespoon safflower oil (or your favorite hair oil)
1 tablespoon shea butter (melted)

Instructions

1. Add the clay and marshmallow root powder to a medium sized bowl. Whisk the clay and marshmallow root powder. Make sure any lumps or clumps are removed. We don't want to wash these out of our hair!
2. Pour aloe vera juice in with the clay and powder. Stir until everything is mixed together.
3. Stir in honey and safflower oil.

4. If your mixture is too dry, add more aloe vera juice by tablespoon. Continue to stir all of the ingredients by hand to reach the consistency you like.
5. This is also a great mix to use after you've worn braids or twists for a few weeks (or months) and want to deeply cleanse your hair and scalp.

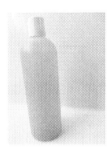

Chelating Cactus Syrup

#3 Chelating Cactus Syrup

If you check the back of your favorite shampoos, you might see the secret ingredient in this recipe—EDTA. EDTA (ethylene diamine tetra-acetic acid) is a chelating agent most known for removing heavy metals and minerals from cosmetics. It keeps your products, hair, scalp, and skin fresh.

When used in DIY hair cleansers, EDTA removes soap scum that can develop over time from hard water. It also lifts and grabs onto heavy metals, removing them from hair and skin. This gives hair a clean, fresh feel and a healthy glow. This is a great recipe to use after wearing a protective style (braids, twists) for some time.

Calcium EDTA

I use calcium EDTA as part of chelation therapy with our son, Damon. Chelation therapy is used as a treatment for heavy metal toxicity in humans. We've used it for a few years to remove heavy metals like arsenic, cadmium, mercury, copper, and more from his bloodstream.

Chelation therapy has helped restore health, wellness, and joy to his system. It's also the absolute best for getting chlorine out of your hair in minutes, without leaving your hair feeling stripped.

You can find EDTA online in powder form and in capsules. You don't need much. This recipe will cleanse, soften, and detox your hair from heavy metals, chlorine, and negative energy.

Chelating Cactus Syrup Recipe

16-ounce bottle with top
2 cactus (nopales) leaves (peeled and cleaned)
4 cups of distilled water
1/8 teaspoon (500 mg) calcium disodium EDTA

Instructions

1. Chop each cactus leaf into four pieces. Cactus leaf may also be listed as Nopales in your local grocery store.
2. Grate each piece until it becomes green mush.
3. Place grated cactus into a large bowl.
4. Add 4 cups of distilled water
5. Cover and let sit for 4 hours.
6. The water will thicken as it sits.
7. Strain cactus leaves from the syrup and throw them away.
8. Add in calcium disodium EDTA to the syrup and stir.
9. Pour the syrup into your bottle.

How To Use:

Apply a handful to wet hair and work through your hair from the scalp, to your ends. Once your hair is saturated, rinse until the syrup is gone. Store unused chelating cactus syrup in your refrigerator for up to 3 weeks.

Note

Do not eat or drink calcium EDTA or EDTA in any form without being under the supervision of a medical doctor or health care professional.

For a natural chelating agent, eat and drink more cilantro. Cilantro is a powerful, all-natural blood cleanser that can remove heavy metals from the bloodstream.

#4 Hair Detox | Cherry Club Soda

Cherries are nature's natural vitamin for hair, skin, and nails! Eating a bowl of cherries can boost your immune system, give you healthy, vibrant skin, and reduce your risk of cancer.

This recipe takes a naturally detoxifying club soda and adds hair-softening, revitalizing cherry pulp to the mix. Cherry pulp hydrates the scalp, prevents dandruff, and adds volume to your hair. It also helps balance the pH levels of hair and skin.

Other benefits of cherries include:

- *improves circulation*
- *helps with weight loss*
- *freshens hair and scalp*
- *causes hair growth in balding areas*
- *has a calming effect on the mind and body*
- *helps prevent weakening of the heart and nervous system (making it a powerful antiaging food)*
- *prevents the growth and spread of cancer cells*
- *induces and improves the quality of sleep*
- *relieves moodiness and anxiety*
- *strengthens brain function*
- *improves memory*

- *reduces stress*
- *repairs damaged hair follicles*
- *provides nourishment and nutrients to the scalp*

Note

Black cherries have a better effect on hair loss and recovery. Montmorency (tart) cherries have been found to help the body recover better and faster[5], especially after exercise.[11]

Cherry Club Soda Recipe

Ingredients

1 bottle of club soda
1 cup fresh cherries

Instructions

1. Remove the seeds from the cherries.
2. Blend cherries and 1/4 cup of the club soda until well mixed.
3. Pour the cherry club soda mixture and remaining club soda into 2-quart pitcher.
4. Pour over your hair for an anytime detox.
5. Rinse out well and follow up with your favorite conditioner.

Optional:

Dip your fingers into the pulp mixture and gently massage it into your scalp. Allow this mixture to sit on your scalp for 10 minutes.

#5 Lavishly Natural's Herbal Shampoo

When my kids were little, this was the only thing I used to wash their hair! It doesn't dry out the skin and it's made with ingredients you know. The calendula flower softens and helps control frizz, the rosemary stimulates hair growth, and the lavender works as a natural conditioner. This is recipe great for kids and naturalistas with sensitive skin.

Ingredients

16-ounce bottle with sealable top
16 ounces distilled water
2 tablespoons calendula flower
2 tablespoons rosemary
2 tablespoons lavender
1/3 cup liquid castile soap
2 teaspoons avocado oil
25 drops lavender oil
25 drops lemon oil

Instructions

1. Bring distilled water to a boil. Add in the calendula, rosemary, and lavender flowers. Reduce to low heat and cover.
2. Let the flowers simmer for 20 minutes.
3. Strain the calendula, rosemary, and lavender from the water and discard the flowers. Allow the water to cool for 5 minutes.
4. Gently add in your castile soap, avocado oil, lavender oil, and lemon oil.
5. Pour the shampoo into your bottle.
6. Shake well before using.
7. You can substitute your own essential oils in this recipe.

#6 Laila's Conditioning Curly Clay Wash

Doing hair at our home salon is not something my little girl enjoys. Not. One. Bit. Luckily, I can cleanse, condition, detangle, and strengthen her curls with one recipe — this one!

Laila's Conditioning Curly Clay Wash is packed with our fave bentonite clay, and her superpower friends:

- *Apple Cider Vinegar* - clarifies and cleanses
- *Marshmallow Root Powder* - conditions, detangles, adds slip to your recipe; makes your recipe easier to rinse out
- *Rhassoul Clay* - conditions, elongates curls
- *Amla Powder* - conditions, intensifies curl definition
- *Safflower Oil* - nourishes the scalp and hair shaft
- *Cocoa Butter* - actually a wax, heals the skin, gives hair more moisture and shine
- *Shea Butter* - heals scalp and skin, keeps hair from drying out
- *Water or Aloe Vera Juice* - hyrdates scalp and skin

Ingredients

1/4 cup bentonite clay
1/2 cup apple cider vinegar
3 tablespoons honey
2 tablespoons marshmallow root powder
2 tablespoons rhassoul clay
1 tablespoon amla powder
1 tablespoon safflower oil
1 tablespoon cocoa butter
1 tablespoon shea butter
1 cup of grapefruit juice
4 to 6 drops grapefruit essential oil (or use your favorite)
a large mixing bowl
a 16 ounce jar or container with sealable lid

Instructions

1. You can mix this in a bowl or blender.
2. Mix the bentonite clay and vinegar first.
3. Add sunflower oil, honey and lemon essential oil.
4. If it starts to clump up on you, begin adding grapefruit juice. Start with 1/2 cup and continue to add until you reach your desired consistency.
5. Apply it to your hair, let it sit for 30 to 45 minutes, and rinse … well.
6. Sunflower oil substitution: jojoba, castor, coconut, and avocado oils also work well in this recipe.

Now that you have six shampoo recipes to add to your diy collection, let's move to the next phase of our hair washing cycle — conditioning!

Chapter 4

DIY Plant-Based Conditioners That Rock

If you love using aloe vera gel in your hair and skin products, then you'll really love her succulent sister cactus! The gel that comes from fresh cactus is an emulsifier[53] that reduces swelling, inflammation, and split ends. Its natural gelatinous quality makes it wonderful for skin care. You can also use fresh cactus gel as a facial mask that's gentle enough for all skin types.

You may have heard of fenugreek seeds before. They're often suggested as a supplement for breastfeeding mommies who want to increase their milk production.

I've used them for this in the past (and stored months of extra breastmilk:) but it's what it does for hair that got me even more excited! Fenugreek seeds are emulsifying agents[66] that speed hair growth. When added to this conditioner, you're also adding increased thickness to your coily greatness.

Fenugreek seeds are actually legumes that help fight cancer, reduce the effects of diabetes and improves the immune system.[66] With it's sweet syrup smell, fenugreek is used in baking, cooking, and can even be enjoyed as a tea (prevents and calms and upset stomach). Make my recipe @ LavishlyNatural.com/fenugreektea

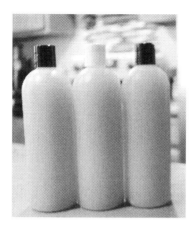

Cactus Fenugreek Conditioner

Ingredients

Cactus Conditioner

1 peeler or small knife
2 large bowls
3 medium cactus leaves (or pads)
4 cups distilled water

Fenugreek Conditioner

2/3 cup fenugreek powder (or fenugreek seeds)
6 cups water
Saran wrap or foil
15 drops lavender essential oil
5 drops sage essential oil
16-ounce bottle with a sealable top

Instructions

1. Cleanse and prep cactus leaves by carefully removing the needles. You can use a peeler for this by peeling the needles off. If you don't have a peeler, use a small knife to cut off the outer layer of the cactus.
2. Cut cactus leaves into four pieces (better for food processing or grating).
3. In a large bowl, grate the leaves into a pulp, or use a food processor.
4. It's okay if pieces are left in the cactus; we're using it all!
5. Add 4 cups of water.
6. Cover with saran wrap or foil and let the cactus conditioner sit for 4 hours.

Make the Fenugreek Conditioner

Instructions

1. While the cactus conditioner sits, start making the fenugreek conditioner. In a large bowl, add the remaining 6 cups of water and fenugreek powder (or fenugreek seeds).
2. Cover this mixture with saran wrap, and let the fenugreek conditioner sit for 4 hours.
3. Both mixtures will thicken a lot.
4. When 4 hours are up, combine the conditioners in the same bowl.
5. Use a strainer, T-shirt, nut milk bag, or scarf to strain the cactus and fenugreek from the Conditioner and discard. *I like to leave these pieces in and blend it all (about 2 minutes) into a hydrating hair smoothie.*
6. After straining or blending your conditioner, add in the lavender and sage essential oils. Gently stir or shake the conditioner to blend in the oils.
7. Apply conditioner to hair and scalp. Condition for 20 minutes. Rinse and style.
8. Add remaining conditioner to bottle with a sealable top. Store in the refrigerator for up to 3 weeks.

Coco Vanilla Leave-In Conditioner

Ingredients

1 cup distilled or purified water
1 teaspoon flax oil
3 to 5 drops vanilla essential oil (or essential of your choice)
1/4 teaspoon guar gum
1/4 teaspoon xanthan gum
1 tablespoon organic coconut oil
Optional liquid substitute: 1 cup coconut milk

Instructions

1. Pour water into a high-speed blender. Add guar gum and xanthan gum to blender.
2. Blend on high speed for up to 2 minutes.
3. Add in flax oil, coconut oil, and vanilla essential oil.
4. Blend for about 30 seconds.
5. For a deeper condition, substitute warm coconut milk for the water

Creamy Avocado Deep Conditioner

Ingredients

2 tablespoons honey
1 ripe avocado (or 1/2 cup mashed)
1 teaspoon fresh lemon juice
1/4 cup aloe vera juice
1 teaspoon castor oil

Instructions

1. Add honey, avocado, and lemon juice to your mixing bowl or blender.
2. Blend for 1 to 2 minutes or until the conditioner reaches your desired consistency. Slowly add in aloe vera juice and castor oil.
3. Increase the aloe vera juice if your conditioner is too thick. Add more avocado if your mix is too thin.

Notes

For over-the-top lavish abundance (and if you have an aloe vera plant), use the natural gel that comes from the leaves of the plant. You may also substitute coconut milk for aloe vera juice for an even creamier avocado conditioner!

Hair Milk

http://lavishlynatural.com/hairmilk/

I love using thick, creamy products in my hair, but there are times when it goes through detox periods and wants nothing milky, creamy, or creamy-ish in her coils. *That's when I pull out the big seeds—flaxseeds!*

Two tablespoons of flaxseeds contain 133 percent of omega-3 fatty acids. Omega-3s are wonderful for our hair, brain, body, and immune system. These EFAs cleanse the arteries, support the heart, boost immune-system function, and nourish the brain (pg. 22, Gladstar, 2001).

You don't have to eat this recipe for your hair to experience the softening, healthy hair-growth wonders of flaxseeds. But … if you would like a recipe you can eat, try my Sweet Flax Milk. It's really good! Mix 1 cup with a teaspoon of flax oil, and it makes a wonderful deep-conditioning hair rinse.

Hair Milk Recipe

Ingredients

2 1/2 cups water
1/4 cup flaxseeds
1 teaspoon aloe vera gel
1 tablespoon coconut oil
2 to 4 drops your favorite essential (palmarosa essential oil goes well in this recipe:)

Instructions

1. Bring flaxseeds to a boil, then reduce to medium-high heat for 10 to 15 minutes.
2. After boiling, strain the flaxseeds out of your gel quickly. It will be thickening as you pour.

3. After you've poured the flaxseed gel into a bowl, add the aloe vera gel, essential oils, and coconut oil.
4. I like to stir this recipe, but you can also use a blender/mixer on low to medium speed for up to 1 minute.
5. This recipe will last up to 3 weeks. Keep it stored in your refrigerator.

Note

The coconut oil in this recipe gives it that creamy look and feel without being oily or greasy. It also won't clog your pores.

Strengthen Your Hair with a Banana Smoothie

Bananas are deeply moisturizing, conditioning, and naturally softening to your luscious hair and skin. When combined with Vitamin B5 (panthenol), it makes a strengthening hair mask that stops and prevents hair breakage and shedding.

Bananas are packed with lots of vitamins and minerals including:

- **Potassium** (422.44 percent—lowers your risk of heart disease and prevents plaque buildup in the arteries)
- **Vitamin B6** (25 percent—prevents insomnia, reduces irritability, balances mood)
- **Vitamin C** (14 percent—prevents skin wrinkling)
- **Manganese** (16 percent—a mineral that controls blood sugar, alleviates PMS)
- **Biotin** (10 percent—supports the health of the skin, nerves, digestive tract, metabolism, and cells)
- **Fiber** (12 percent—decreases your risk of stroke, improves weight loss)
- **Copper** (10 percent—gives you energy, helps maintain blood volume, helps balance cholesterol)

Conditioning with Vitamin B5

Panthenol is a water-soluble nutrient from the B vitamin family that's very hygroscopic *(absorbs moisture from the air)*. This powerful humectant is used as D-panthenol in hair-care products and cosmetics.[71]

Panthenol benefits include:

- *moisturizing*
- *penetrates the skin*
- *helps in tissue repair*
- *natural hair strengthener*
- *helps speed the healing of wounds*
- *conditions hair without buildup*
- *adds suppleness to skin*
- *non-irritating skin softener*
- *protects the skin against sunburn*[53]

Note

I add between 1/8 teaspoon to 1/4 teaspoon of panthenol to my flaxseed jellies, leave-ins, hair teas, tonics, and conditioners. This gives my hair an instant power boost without the crunchiness.

Less is best when testing this panthenol in your handmade products. Even one to two drops can be enough. If your hair loves vitamin B5 treatments, consider adding panthenol to your natural hair-care regime.

Banana-Nilla Vitamin B5 Hair Smoothie

1 ripe banana (blended)
3 tablespoons raw honey
1/2 cup Greek yogurt
2 tablespoons raw apple cider vinegar
1/8 teaspoon DL panthenol
3 drops vanilla essential oil (or your favorite)

Instructions

1. Add banana, honey, yogurt, apple cider vinegar, panthenol and vanilla essential oil to a bowl or blender.
2. Stir until ingredients are mixed together and smooth. If using a blender, blend for up to 1 minute.
3. Apply to the ends of your hair.
4. Let condition 20 to 45 minutes.
5. I like to leave mine on for the day, but test this recipe on your hair to see how long works wonderfully for you!
6. Rinse and style!

Recipe Extra: Something You Can Drink | Mulberry Banana Smoothie

Ingredients

1 banana
1 1/2 cup coconut milk (rice milk and sweet flax milk are great substitutes)
1 teaspoon maple syrup
1 tablespoon fresh mulberries
1 teaspoon lucema powder
1 teaspoon vanilla
a handful of ice
Optional Awesomeness: 1 teaspoon matcha green tea

Instructions

1. Add all of the ingredients into a high-speed blender. Blend until smooth.
2. Pour it into a glass and drink expeditiously!

Raw Banana Conditioning Hair Mask

Ingredients

4 ripe bananas
1/2 teaspoon fresh lemon juice
1 tablespoon apricot kernel oil
1 teaspoon raw agave syrup (or molasses)

Instructions

1. Add the bananas, lemon juice, apricot kernel oil, and agave syrup to a high-speed blender.
2. Blend all of the ingredients for up to 1 minute in the blender, or until the mix is the consistency of a smoothie.
3. This recipe makes 16 ounces.
4. Apply to your hair and let condition for up to 20 minutes.
5. Rinse and style.
6. Use within 7 days. Keep stored in your refrigerator.

Notes

Naturally detangles hair and leaves it shiny and well moisturized. The smoothie texture makes it easy to rinse right out. If you're using firm bananas, it may be an issue. Blend them for an extra two minutes or until smooth.

DIY Conditioning Hair Smoothie

Ingredients

1/2 cup coconut milk
1 tablespoon olive oil
2 tablespoons honey
4 drops vanilla essential oil

Instructions

1. In this recipe, you can always substitute your favorite essential oil or leave it out all together.
2. Mix or blend all your ingredients for about 2 minutes for a slightly thicker smoothie consistency.
3. Apply the smoothie to wet hair.
4. Leave it on for 30 to 45 minutes.
5. Rinse and style.

Note

Because it contains oil, you can apply heat for an even deeper conditioning experience (hair dryer, heat cap). I usually put my hair in a baggie and let body heat do its thing!

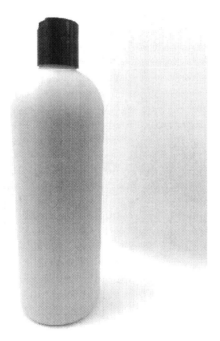

Fenugreek Smoothie

Coconut Cream Smoothie (for Hair)

This Coconut Cream Smoothie:

- *is a great detangler (it has the perfect amount of slip) on dry or wet hair*
- *requires less than two minutes to make (but six hours to get ready)*
- *will grow your hair (with noticeable results) within 30 days*

Bold claims right?

This smoothie helped stop the thinning drama at my crown completely. It was the fenugreek! This recipe calls for a little less than a cup of these syrup smelling seeds. When applied regularly to the scalp, fenugreek seeds:

- *enhance hair growth and regrowth*
- *decrease hair thinning*
- *stop hair loss*

The slippery elm bark is optional in the recipe, but it gives it such a great creamy feel. It's also the ingredient that turns your leftover fenugreek smoothie into a conditioning pudding. It has the texture of a pudding and goes on like a cream. This recipe will last in the refrigerator for up to six weeks. Just stir it before using.

Coconut Cream Smoothie

Ingredients

1/2 cup fenugreek seeds (whole or powdered)
4 cups distilled water
2 tablespoons slippery elm bark powder
2 tablespoons coconut cream
1 teaspoon coconut oil

Instructions

1. Add seeds or powder to distilled water.
2. Soak the seeds for 6 hours.
3. After soaking, strain the seeds from the water and set them to the side. Pour the water into a separate bowl.
4. Add the seeds and 1 cup of fenugreek water to a high-speed blender.
5. Blend for 2 minutes.
6. Add coconut cream and coconut oil. Blend for 30 seconds.
7. Massage the coconut cream smoothie into the scalp and condition for 20 to 30 minutes.
8. Rinse thoroughly and style!

Food-Based Substitutions for Coconut Cream

If you don't have coconut cream, try some of these substitutions. Use 2 tablespoons of any of the following:

- avocado (mashed and pureed)
- bananas (mashed and pureed)
- coconut butter
- honey
- molasses
- maple syrup
- raw agave syrup

Hard Water Alternatives

I like to save the water the fenugreek seeds make for hair rinses. You may want to add more liquid to your smoothie or pudding. If you're looking for hard water alternatives, try these:

- *distilled water*
- *aloe vera juice*
- *cactus gel*
- *green tea*
- *hibiscus tea*
- *fenugreek hair rinse*
- *flaxseed water*
- *rose water*
- *club soda*
- *2 tablespoons apple cider vinegar in 2 cups water*

Chapter 5

8 Hair Teas That Are Better Than Your Creamiest Conditioner

It was the summer of 2015. I had just gotten the swing of the water only hair washing method, and loving the fact that water (and coconut water, and cactus syrup, and shea butter, and...) and other ingredients, were keeping my hair healthy and happy.

That's when I picked up my favorite deep conditioner. I put it on as usual, let it stay on my hair the desired amount of time (about an hour), and rinsed. It was like I had a white paste on my hair and the more I tried to wash it out, the worse it became.

My hair was revolting against creamy conditioners, and styling creams.

My buttery goodness, thicky thick deep conditioners would all of the sudden stop penetrating, and start sitting...right on top of my hair. Maybe it was the hard water, maybe it was the pool, maybe it was santa, but my hair didn't care. Since lavish cannot go without conditioner, I set out on a natural quest for conditioners that wouldn't leave product buildup, but were equally as conditioning.

Here are eight of the best!

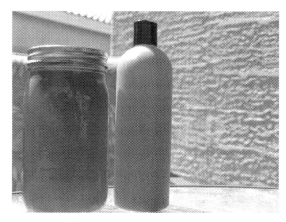

Hibiscus Hair Tea Ingredients

#1 Hibiscus Hair Tea

This recipe comes from my 2015 Summer DIY Collection. It's our most popular hair tea recipe ever, and I know why … it's super-conditioning! I know what you're thinking: *It's a hair tea, how conditioning can it be?*

It could be the deep conditioning power of the catnip or the hair-healing properties of comfrey root. Hibiscus flowers are deeply conditioning. When applied to your hair, hibiscus helps heal the scalp, balance mood, and unblocks creativity.

Hibiscus flowers will turn your recipes a slight red color. This red flower power helps balance your root chakra, which means you'll feel more safe, secure, and deeply connected to life.

Oh, and did I say it adds shine to your hair?

Try using it as a rinse, hair spritz, or leave-in. For the other recipes in the Summer DIY Collection, see the Organic Hair Butter (pg. 83) and Homemade Sunscreen (http://lavishlynatural.com/sunscreen/)

Ingredients

2 tablespoons fresh or dried hibiscus flowers

2 tablespoons dandelion root

2 tablespoons flaxseeds

3 sprigs rosemary leaves (or 10 drops of rosemary essential oil)

8 cups water

2 tablespoons catnip flower

1 tablespoon comfrey root 2 (16-ounce) bottles or a 32-ounce jar with top

Instructions

1. Add hibiscus, dandelion root, flaxseeds, and rosemary leaves to water.
2. Bring to a boil.
3. Turn heat to low and simmer for 5 minutes.
4. Remove from heat and let sit for 5 minutes.
5. Add catnip and comfrey root to warm water and let sit for 10 minutes.
6. Strain leaves, flowers, and seeds from water and discard.
7. Pour into bottles.
8. Keep in refrigerator for up to two months.

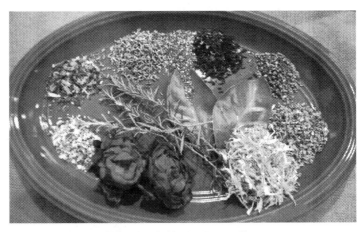

Hibiscus Hair Tea Ingredients

Go Lavishly Natural

Hibiscus Hair Tea Ingredient Benefits

Catnip – can be used in place of conditioner; moisturizes hair; heals split ends; increases hair volume and thickness

Comfrey root – stimulates the scalp; heals scalp irritations; speeds wound healing; stimulates hair growth; softens hair; prevents hair loss

Dandelion root – tones the skin; helps balance sebum in the scalp, which promotes hair growth; relieves dandruff

Roses – fragrant; extremely rich in flavonoids and vitamins A, C, D, E, and B3; a natural moisturizer that rejuvenates hair

Hibiscus flower – can be used as a natural hair dye; has a high mucilage content, making it a wonderful hair and skin moisturizer that is gentle for sensitive skin; helps hair and skin retain moisture

Lavender flower – a cleansing oil that prevents hair loss; a cell rejuvenator that prevents scarring and stretch marks; a balancing flower/oil that relaxes and stimulates

Calendula flowers – works as a natural emollient; soothes scalp irritation; a cell rejuvenator that helps hair follicles grow, creating thicker hair

Rosemary leaves – improve circulation and blood flow to the scalp; help prevent and treat hair loss; prevent baldness; aid in hair growth

Lemon leaves – rich in antioxidants and vitamins, which are beneficial for perfect skin, hair, and health

Chia seeds – packed with vitamins A, B, C, copper, and iron; restore health and strength to hair; rich in omega-3 fatty acids, prevent hair loss; give hair luster and shine

Flaxseed – high in omega-3s; revitalizes the skin; nourishes the hair and scalp; adds shine; softens the hair; helps define curls

#2 Catty Comfrey Conditioner

I have a really, really deep love for creamy conditioners. Aubrey Organics Honeysuckle Rose, Island Naturals, and Blue Chamomile conditioners were part of my deep-conditioning team for years.

That was until I got catty.

I had read about the benefits of catnip for hair, and since I don't have cats (I hear it can get them pretty excited), I thought it would be safe to try. I was looking for a recipe I could use on my girls' hair while they were learning to swim. Swim class was once a week, and the chlorinated water wasn't mixing well with the creamy conditioners.

We could still deep condition monthly, just not following each swim session. We needed something that had the same conditioning power but less buildup, oil, and greasiness. I had been using catnip for hair growth with success and decided to use it as a rinse after swimming. It worked so well we started using it as a leave-in spritz to keep twists fresh and moisturized.

It's been three years and we haven't looked back!

Ingredient Spotlight: Catnip

Once catnip is heated, it will release its essential oils. These oils lightly coat the hair shaft, giving your hair a fuller, softer look and feel.

The benefits of catnip include:

- *heals and prevents split ends*
- *moisturizes and conditions hair*
- *works as a hair lightener*
- *skin toner, natural astringent (great for sensitive skin)*
- *calms and soothes the body*

- *strengthens hair*
- *works great as a leave-in conditioner and spritz*

The other main ingredient I add to this recipe is comfrey root. Comfrey root is a medicinal herb that works as a natural emollient for your hair.

Comfrey root is also great for:

- *new cell growth*
- *reducing inflammation*
- *healing wounds, scars*
- *helping maintain healthy skin*

I add a handful of hibiscus flowers (I add a handful of them to everything) for shine and extra conditioning, but this is optional. Catnip tea is great all by itself.

Catty Comfrey Conditioner Recipe

Ingredients

4 cups hot water
2 tablespoons dried catnip
1 tablespoon dried comfrey root
*Optional: handful of dried hibiscus flowers

Instructions

1. Add the ingredients to hot water.
2. Let it sit for 5 minutes.
3. Strain the herbs from the water and discard the herbs.
4. Use as a deep conditioning hair rinse, pre-poo (used before you cleanse your hair, usually on dry hair), or daily hair spritz.

#3 Dandelion Hair Tea

When I was little, the first bouquet of flowers I made for myself was a big bunch of yellow dandelions from the yard. Very few things were better than blowing dandelions in the wind and pretending they were snow (it never snowed in Nashville).

I had no idea that you could boil those suckers and drink them for an extremely healthy tea that's even more magical for your hair! Dandelions are an edible herb packed with healing vitamins and minerals.

Dandelion tea benefits include:

- *it's power packed with the following vitamins and minerals: iron, zinc, calcium, potassium, copper, and vitamins A, B, C, and D[4]*
- *natural skin toner*
- *natural laxative*
- *natural diuretic,[16, 36]*
- *settles an upset stomach, helps ease digestion*
- *relieves bloating*
- *purifies the blood[15]*
- *helps control blood sugar*
- *often used to treat cancer, viral infections[17]*
- *reduces inflammation*
- *cleanses the liver*
- *relieves dandruff*
- *gives great hair sheen (a cousin to hair shine)*
- *helps control acne, diabetes, and high blood pressure*
- *helps balance the sebum in your scalp, which promotes hair growth*
- *relieves dry hair*

The tea itself can be pretty bitter, so make sure to use your favorite sweetener. Stevia and honey are great options.

Note:

For naturalistas with allergies or sensitive skin: do not use this recipe if you have a ragweed allergy or if you are allergic to chrysanthemums, daisies, or marigolds.

Dandelion Hair Tea Recipe

2 1/2 cups of water
1 tablespoon (or 1 tea bag) dandelion root
2 tablespoons of flaxseeds
1 tablespoon honey
5 drops lemon essential oil (or 1 teaspoon lemon juice)
*optional: 1 to 2 teaspoons apple cider vinegar
20-ounce bottle

Instructions

1. Seep your dandelion root or dandelion root tea bag in 1 cup of water for 4 to 5 minutes.
2. Strain dandelion root from water if using scoops. Set dandelion tea to the side.
3. Boil flaxseeds in 1 1/2 cups of water for 4 to 5 minutes.
4. Remove from heat and strain the flaxseeds from the water immediately.
5. Add honey to hot flaxseed water (consistency should be slippery) and allow the mixture to cool for 10 minutes.
6. Combine dandelion tea, flaxseed water, apple cider vinegar, and lemon in 20-ounce bottle.
7. Shake to get all of the ingredients happy and blended.
8. Wash and condition your hair. Pour the tea over your hair for your final rinse.
9. Let it sit on your gorgeous curls for 5 to 10 minutes. Cover your hair with a plastic cap for a deeper condition.
10. Rinse and style!

#4 Dandelion and Hibiscus Hair Tea

This conditioning tea helps prevent split ends and keeps your hair hydrated. The nourishing flaxseeds give it a little slip that also helps keep frizz down. The hibiscus gives this recipe a deep conditioning, hair growth boost.

Ingredients

4 cups water (32 ounces)
1 tablespoon dried hibiscus (will turn your tea red)
1 tablespoon dandelion tea
2 tablespoons catnip tea
2 tablespoons comfrey root
1 tablespoon flaxseeds
1/4 cup aloe vera juice
4 drops lemon essential oil (or your favorite essential oil)

Instructions

1. Bring water to a boil.
2. Add hibiscus and remove from heat.
3. Add dandelion tea, catnip tea, comfrey root, and flaxseeds.
4. Let cool for 15 minutes.
5. Add aloe vera juice.
6. Add four drops of lemon essential oil (or your favorite) for fragrance.

Note

Add this conditioner to the end of your hair-washing routine for best results. You can leave it on your hair for 5 to 10 minutes for deep conditioning before rinsing. *Place your hair under a plastic cap and use your body heat for a hot tea treatment!*

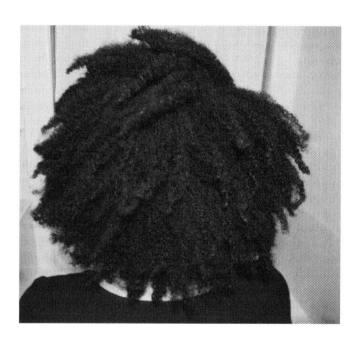

#5 Lavishly Natural Slippery Marshmallow Detangling Conditioner

If you've ever enjoyed the slippery-ness of a good, slippery detangler, you may already be familiar with marshmallow root. Marshmallow root powder comes from the beautiful marshmallow plant (Althaea officinalis). You may also see it referred to as *althea extract*, *marshmallow extract*, and *marshmallow root extract*.

It's roots and leaves are used to:

- *heal the skin*
- *reduce inflammation*
- *get rid of congestion*
- *add soothing slip and softness to hair*
- *make marshmallows (and top off a good cup of hot chocolate)*

Consumed mostly as a tea, marshmallow root is what gives some of your favorite natural hair products their trademark slip, which can shorten any detangling regime.

It is sold as a vitamin, extract, tea, or powder (and you can buy it in bulk:). I prefer using the powder form because it lasts forever, and it's easier to measure. I use marshmallow root powder for its slip factor, and also for its super natural thickening and conditioning powers.

Make Your Light Conditioners A Little Thicker

Like xanthan gum and guar gum, which also thicken soups and sauces, marshmallow root will thicken anything it's added to. Homemade shampoos, conditioners, teas, hair smoothies, hair milk — almost any diy recipe you can think of. Think along the lines of a more firming flaxseed gel but even more soft and slippery.

This is orgasmic for homemade conditioners, moisturizers, and any of your water-based goodies. I even add it to all of my clay mixes to help absorb liquid (if I add too much) and to make the treatment easier to rinse out.

This bodacious botanical also makes an excellent aftershave for the naturlistos in your life. Luscious hubby uses it for this and as a gentle conditioner for his sexy skin.

Marshmallow Root Benefits

- has emollient, soothing, and healing capabilities when incorporated into skin-care formulations
- beneficial in aftershave preparations and in products that treat sunburns and dry skin
- natural hydroglycolic plant extract from the althea root
- pain relieving
- works as an anti-itching agent

Lavishly Natural's Slippery Marshmallow Detangling Conditioner Recipe

Ingredients

3 cups purified water, divided
2 tablespoons catnip
2 tablespoons marshmallow root powder
1 tablespoon apple cider vinegar
grapefruit essential oil (or your favorites)

Instructions

1. Heat 2 cups of water to just before boiling and remove from heat.
2. Add catnip and let it sit for 10 minutes.
3. Strain catnip roots/leaves from the water and discard.
4. Bring the remaining cup of water to a boil.

5. Add marshmallow root powder and apple cider vinegar to boiling water.
6. Remove from heat. Allow it to cool for 10 to 15 minutes.
7. Add catnip-infused water to marshmallow root/apple cider mixture. Add essential oils and have a lavish hair partay!

How To Use

Gently rinse your hair after use. This recipe is great for use after shampoo, co-wash (washing your hair with conditioner, no shampoo), and deep conditioner. Also good as a hair rinse.

Recipe Extra | Marshmallow Root Conditioner

A popular marshmallow root recipe suggested by *Lavishly Natural Readers*, is this simple marshmallow root conditioner.

Ingredients

a 32 ounce bottle or jar, with sealable top,
1 cup of marshmallow root powder,
and 3 cups of purified water.

Instructions

1. Add one cup of marshmallow root powder (or dried leaves and stems) to three cups of hot purified water.
2. Pour this conditioner mix into your blender and blend on high speed for 1 minute. You may need to work this conditioner through your hair with your fingers.
3. Leave it on for about 20 minutes and rinse.

#6 Flower Therapy | Rose Water Replenishing Hair Tonic

This recipe comes from weeding my garden and needing something to do with the roses and rosemary that had fallen to the ground. Just the right ingredients to inspire a hair tonic that naturally smells like roses, and keeps your hair and skin happy.

Ingredients

1 cup distilled water
1/4 cup dried organic red or pink roses
1 tablespoon dried organic hibiscus flowers
1 1/2 cups flaxseed water (2 tablespoons of flaxseeds in 1 1/2 cup of distilled water)
4 to 6 drops rose essential oil
4 to 6 drops sandalwood essential oil
optional: fresh or dried rosemary and mint

Instructions

1. In a small pot, bring distilled water, roses, and hibiscus to a boil and immediately reduce heat. Let simmer on low to low-medium heat for 15 minutes. Remove from heat to cool.
2. In a separate pot, bring flaxseeds and water to a boil for 4 to 5 minutes.
3. Immediately pour flaxseed water through a strainer to remove all flaxseeds.
4. Strain the flowers out of your rose water and discard.
5. Add rose water to flaxseed water and pour into your bottle(s).
6. This mix is enough for two 8-ounce bottles or one mega 16-ounce bottle for a concentrated dose of softening, conditioning power!

Recipe Notes

Make sure to store your flaxseeds in an airtight container. They will last about three weeks in the refrigerator, and you can reuse them at least one to two more times for fresh flaxseed water and gel!

Lavish option: Add one sprig of fresh rosemary and one sprig of fresh mint to the flaxseed liquid before boiling for a natural infusion of botanical goodness!

Recipe Extras

Revitalizing Hair Tonic: Add 1 tablespoon of aloe vera juice and 1 teaspoon of vegetable glycerin to the Rosy Thoughts Mind Cleanser recipe, and it becomes a nourishing hair tonic! The vegetable glycerin will give this tonic a teeny-tiny bit of slip that acts like a moisture magnet for your hair. It also keeps this tonic oil-free. Optional: if frizz is a concern, add 1/2 teaspoon of calendula extract to eliminate frizz completely!

Don't Like Glycerin in Your DIY Products?

Try using fresh cactus syrup mixed with calendula extract instead. The cactus syrup will give hair a nice slip like the glycerin with extra hydrating benefits. The calendula extract acts as an emollient that softens, moisturizes, and nourishes hair and skin.

Rose Sandalwood Replenishing Hair Tonic is wonderful to use as a rinse or leave-in spritz.

Bonus Recipe: DIY Rose Water

The next time you receive roses, don't throw them out when they start to dry. Take the whole flower or rose petals and add them to one cup of water. Turn the water on low heat and let it simmer for up to 30 minutes.

Strain the roses out of the water and allow it to cool. Makes about 6 ounces of rose water.

Ingredient Spotlight | Rose Water Replenishing Hair Tonic

Organic red or pink roses – soften and condition the hair; promote hair growth; help hair maintain proper balance of moisture

Organic hibiscus flowers – great for scalp stimulation and hair conditioning; adds fullness and thickens the hair

Flaxseed water – adds natural slip and shine to thirsty tresses; gives you all of the benefits and moisturizing effects of an oil without being an oil

Rose essential oil – adds a light natural fragrance and transformative mood lifter; boosts self-esteem and confidence

Sandalwood essential oil – grounds the senses; activates a calm, clear mind; natural fragrance; excellent spritz for protective styles, especially easy braids and twists

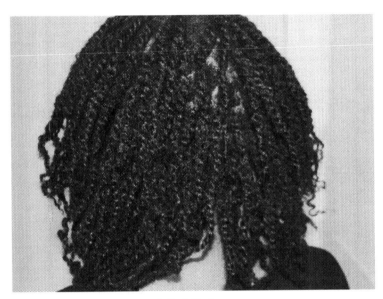

Mini Twists

#7 Lavishly Natural's Luscious Hair Tea

3 cups purified water

1 tablespoon flaxseeds

1 tablespoon chamomile flowers (or 1 tea bag of chamomile tea)

1 tablespoon dried lavender flowers

1/4 cup aloe vera juice

6 drops rose essential oil

optional: 1/8 teaspoon optiphen

Instructions

1. Bring water to a boil.
2. Reduce heat to medium-low and add flaxseeds, chamomile,* and lavender flowers.
3. Simmer for 5 minutes on medium-low heat.
4. Add aloe vera juice and reduce heat to low.
5. Simmer tea for 10 minutes.
6. Remove from heat and add essential oil.
7. Strain leaves and flowers from the tea and allow it to cool.
8. Pour into container or 16-ounce bottle.
9. Apply after wash and condition as a leave-in hair rinse.

*May substitute green tea for chamomile flowers (1 tea bag is enough).

Chamomile flowers:

- smell awesome
- stimulate hair growth
- prevent hair loss
- soften skin

Lavender flowers are naturally hydrating and nourishing to the skin. Researchers have found these flowers to be an effective treatment for alopecia areata (hair loss).[55]

#8 Tea Therapy

Ingredients

2 1/2 cups purified water
1 teaspoon flaxseeds
1 tablespoon dried catnip
1 tablespoon dried comfrey root
1 tablespoon hibiscus flowers
1 teaspoon dried rosemary or 4 drops of rosemary essential oil
optional: 1 teaspoon raw apple cider vinegar

Instructions

1. Bring water to a boil and add flaxseeds. Immediately remove from heat.
2. Add catnip, comfrey root, hibiscus, and rosemary.
3. Let sit for 10 minutes.
4. Strain ingredients from the water and discard.
5. Add apple cider vinegar and rosemary.
6. Remove from heat.

Notes

Great for use after a swim to help rebalance your hair's pH levels. Use as a hair rinse after a shampoo, co-wash, or deep conditioner.

Now that you have recipes for all-natural shampoos and hair teas that cleanse, moisturize, and condition, let's explore recipes that strengthen, clarify and add shine. It's time to talk about it — apple cider vinegar, naturalista gold.

Why is apple cider vinegar so popular for natural hair and body care? Should you add it to your natural regime?

Chapter 6

Vivacious Vinegar Recipes for Healthy, Natural Hair

Most naturalistas have an Apple Cider Vinegar (ACV) Rinse in their rotation at some point. It cleanses, helps clarify, removes product buildup, and leaves luscious shine behind. ACV is best for oily hair, but did you know that rice wine vinegar is milder and better for dry hair?[37] Here are three healthy hair vinegar recipes to add to your collection.

Asia's Apple Cider Vinegar Rinse

I really, really love apple cider vinegar (ACV). I use it to make homemade clay washes, in most of my hair teas, and as a quick scalp cleanser when wearing protective styles. Raw apple cider vinegar (contains the mother) and holds the most benefits for natural styles.

ACV Hair Benefits

- ✓ works as a hair conditioner
- ✓ helps hair retain moisture
- ✓ removes product buildup without stripping the hair of its natural oils
- ✓ balances your pH levels
- ✓ a natural hair cleanser
- ✓ adds shine and reduces frizz

- ✓ reduces tangles
- ✓ helps prevent hair loss
- ✓ itchy dry scalp treatment
- ✓ removes hair lice

Asia's Apple Cider Vinegar Rinse Recipe

Ingredients

4 drops rosemary essential oil
4 drops basil essential oil
4 drops lavender essential oil
2 1/2 cups warm water
3 tablespoons apple cider vinegar
1 tablespoon warm honey
1/2 teaspoon aloe vera extract

Instructions:

1. Place 4 or 5 drops of any of the essential oils listed above into 2 ½ cups of warm water.
2. Stir apple cider vinegar, honey, and aloe vera extract into the water.
3. Pour the rinse over your hair before or after shampooing, co-washing, or conditioning. Rinse the conditioner from your hair. I've also used this rinse as a prewash when my hair is really dirty or if it has a lot of product buildup.
4. If you would like extra conditioning, you can leave it in for 3 or 4 minutes.

Notes:

Dried herbs can be substituted in place of the essential oils.

It's as simple as that, and most people have apple cider vinegar right in their cupboards. It's a quick, easy, and inexpensive route to make hair look salon beautiful without the salon price.

Optional: substitute 1/4 cup aloe vera juice in place of aloe vera extract.

Health Benefits of Apple Cider Vinegar

The scientist in me is always searching for evidence-based health uses for everything. It's a habit! Apple cider vinegar is no different. Like most of the natural ingredients that are good for our hair, this one is also best when eaten.

Make a nice vinaigrette with this tasty super food, or go hardcore with a couple of teaspoons in water when you wake up or right before bed. Drinking ACV has a cleansing and detoxifying effect on the body.

Here Are Eleven Other Benefits You May Not Know ...

1. lowers blood glucose levels[45]
2. lowers cholesterol
3. kills and slows the growth of cancer[51]
4. clears acne
5. relieves stiffness
6. can be used as a natural deodorant
7. keeps bugs off your countertops
8. helps you feel full
9. works as a fruit and veggie cleanser
10. gets rid of dandruff
11. lowers blood pressure

I've used all types of apple cider vinegar, but to get many of the health benefits described above, raw, unfiltered apple cider vinegar is the best. There are several versions. Bragg is a popular one, but I often buy the organic, generic version at my local health-food store. Look around, comparison shop, and see which one works best for you. For all my veggie lovers (and juicers), the following is a quick and easy veggie wash that works.

Fruit & Veggie Wash Recipe

EricaKKing.com/veggiewash

Ingredients

2 tablespoons apple cider vinegar
2 tablespoons lemon juice
1 tablespoon baking soda

Instructions

1. Add to water in a sink or large container.
2. Let your produce sit for 30 minutes in cleanser.
3. Keep your goods soaked in the water (you may need to rotate your ingredients).
4. After 30 minutes, remove and rinse ingredients.
5. Brush off any remaining debris with a veggie brush.
6. Store your ingredients.

Recipe Note:

White vinegar may be used in place of apple cider vinegar

Rice Wine Vinegar Rinse

Rice wine vinegar is a milder option compared to apple cider vinegar but just as effective. Perfect for shinier hair and healthy hair growth.

Ingredients

3 tablespoons rice wine vinegar
2 cups water
6 drops bergamot essential oil
optional: 2 tablespoons coconut water
16-ounce bottle

Instructions

1. Bring 2 cups of water to a boil.
2. Remove from heat and allow water to cool for about 10 minutes.
3. Pour in rice wine vinegar, essential oil and optional coconut oil.
4. Pour into a 16-ounce squeeze bottle and apply to hair.
5. Leave it in for 5 to 10 minutes.
6. Rinse and condition, or style.

Chapter 7

Healing Clay Treatments for Gorgeous Natural Hair

Clay recipes are:

- healing to the mind, body, and soul
- perfect for hair growth
- good for preventing and treating hair loss
- effective for all forms of cleansing and detox[24]

When applied to your hair, clay:

- detangles
- conditions
- strengthens
- heals
- stops hair loss in its tracks
- thickens hair
- strengthens your hair's natural curl definition

Bentonite Clay

Bentonite clay is often used in clay packs to pull toxins, infection, and inflammation from the body. Also referred to as Montmorillonite, bentonite clay has been used medicinally to:

- treat ulcers
- reduce inflammation
- heal gastrointestinal irritation, discomfort
- treat infection
- kill human pathogens (bacteria, fungus, or virus that causes disease)[68]
- bind to toxins and remove them from the body
- heal the mind and body at the cellular level

It's Really Not Mud…It's Ash

Bentonite is a generic term that refers to the rocks that come from volcanic ash. Natural, untreated bentonite deposits are mined all over the world. Ten billion tons of bentonite are mined each year making it easy to find and affordable. Thirty-five percent are mined in the United States, with other reserves located in Australia, Italy, India, and China.

Rhassoul Clay

Rhassoul is a mineral-rich clay that comes from the ancient deposits mined deep beneath the Atlas Mountains in Morocco. It's one of the main ingredients in mud wraps and other spa treatments. Rhassoul clay contains more silica and magnesium than bentonite clay, which adds more softness and smoothness to your skin. Rhassoul clay mixed with cocoa butter is a deep conditioning treatment that elongates curls, moisturizes the hair shaft, and heals the scalp. It also strengthens hair and promotes hair growth,

The recipes that follow are excellent for cleansing, conditioning, and detangling your hair. In addition to their numerous health benefits (clays heal the skin, help cure acne), it's the spiritual qualities of clay that make it my favorite treatment for hair loss.

Clay, when applied externally to hair, scalp, and skin, strengthens your clairvoyant (clear seeing), clairaudient (clear listening), claircognizant (clear thinking), and clairsentient (clear sensing) abilities. These abilities sharpen your mental clarity, memory, decision-making skills, coping methods, confidence, and ability to follow through on the Divine Guidance you receive.

Homemade Bentonite Clay Wash

Ingredients

3 tablespoons bentonite clay

2 tablespoons marshmallow root powder

3 tablespoons apple cider vinegar

1 tablespoon safflower oil (jojoba, coconut, and avocado oils will also work)

1 cup of water

3 tablespoons honey (I like a lot in my mix)

4 to 6 drops your favorite essential oil

Instructions

1. Mix clay, marshmallow root powder, and vinegar first.
2. Add sunflower, honey and your favorite essential oil.
3. If it starts to clump up on you, begin adding water. Start with 2 tablespoons and continue to add until you reach your desired consistency.
4. Apply it to your hair, let it sit for 30 to 45 minutes, and rinse ... well.
5. Play with your ingredients. This is a basic recipe; it likes when you add to it!

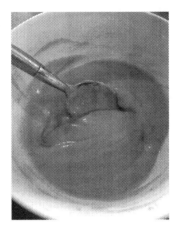

Bentonite Clay Wash

Frankincense & Myrrh Blessed Hair Cleanser

Dry Ingredients

1 cup bentonite clay
1/4 cup alma powder
2 tablespoons rosemary powder
2 tablespoons linden leaf powder
2 tablespoons horsetail powder
1/4 cup marshmallow root powder

Wet Ingredients (add slowly)

1/4 cup honey
2 cups grapefruit juice

Oils and Butters

2 tablespoons castor oil
1/4 cocoa butter (melted)
2 tablespoons shea butter (melted)

Extracts and Essentials

1 teaspoon aloe vera extract
1 teaspoon calendula extract
10 drops frankincense
10 drops myrrh

Instructions

1. Add your dry ingredients to a mixing bowl. Whisk the clay and powders to remove all lumps and clumps. These will show up in your mix and your hair. They are a beast to wash out!
2. Add in apple cider vinegar. Your blend my take on a paste texture. That's okay. Add in grapefruit juice and honey. Clay absorbs liquids extremely well and will thicken as you work with it.
3. Gently melt the cocoa and shea butter if needed. Add butters and oils to your mix and stir.
4. The texture of this recipe is one of a thick smoothie. Add in as much liquid, oils, butters, and extracts as you like. This recipe loves variations and substitutions!

Coconut Milk Clay Conditioner

LavishlyNatural.com/chocolate

This rich, moisturizing rhassoul clay deep conditioner contains high levels of silica, magnesium, and potassium, which are excellent for healthy hair and skin!

Rhassoul clay:

1. *helps remove toxins from hair and body*
2. *softens and conditions hair*
3. *elongates kinky curls*
4. *adds shine*

If you have any leftovers of this recipe, keep them in an air tight container and place it in the refrigerator. If you're using this Chocolate on the same day, saran wrap will work. If you're making a big batch and have lots left over, you can freeze this clay for up to 6 months.

Ingredients

- 3 tablespoons rhassoul clay
- 1/4 cup cocoa butter (*melted, add slowly*)
- 2 tablespoons raw honey
- 2 tablespoons warm coconut milk (or up to 1/2 cup)

Instructions

1. Add all ingredients to your mixing bowl. Stir until the clay is smooth.
2. If you like more of a paste consistency, add less coconut milk. If you like your mix to be more like a thick chocolate sauce (like me:), add more by the teaspoon.

3. Once the clay is mixed, apply it to your hair. Let it condition for 45 to 60 minutes.
4. Rinse well! This clay likes to hide in my coils more than bentonite clay, so make sure to rinse well, then rinse again!
5. Optional: Add a heat cap for a luscious deep condition!

Optional Coconut Milk Substitutions:

Don't have warm coconut milk? Try:

- *aloe vera juice*
- *coconut water*
- *distilled water*
- *grapefruit juice*
- *green tea*
- *homemade flaxseed gel*

Pumpkin Spice Deep-Conditioning Clay Wash

Ingredients

3 tablespoons rhassoul clay
2 tablespoons pumpkin puree
1/4 cup organic cocoa butter
1 teaspoon coconut oil
2 to 3 tablespoons raw or organic honey

optional: 1 teaspoon cacao powder and a dash of cinnamon (or 1/8 teaspoon)
1 cup purified water or your hair's beverage of choice (BOC), which includes:

- coconut milk
- green tea
- aloe vera juice
- coconut water
- flaxseed conditioner (recipe link below)**
- rose water

**_lavishlynatural.com/flaxseed-leave-in-conditioner/_

Instructions

1. Add pumpkin and rhassoul clay to mixing bowl.
2. Melt cocoa butter in the microwave for about 20 seconds or until all pieces are dissolved.
3. Add to clay and pumpkin and mix. Add coconut oil and honey. For an added bit of chocolate conditioning, add 1 teaspoon of organic cacao powder.
4. Heat the liquid until warm (not scalding—leads to unhappy scalp) and add it to the mix. Try to keep from eating it, as it smells wonderful!
5. Place a plastic bag on your hair and let it marinate on your hair for 30 to 45 minutes. Rinse and style as usual.

Recipe Notes

Storage tip: Once you've mixed all the ingredients, you can store this clay in your refrigerator or freezer for months. Simply put it in the refrigerator if you'll be using it in the next few weeks, or freeze it for use a few months from now! When ready to use, take it out of the freezer, let it "warm up" in the refrigerator for a day or so, and that's it.

Erica's Organic Honey Lime Clay Mask (Facial Cleanser)

Ingredients

1/2 teaspoon organic raw honey
1 tablespoon rhassoul clay
1/8 teaspoon collagen
1 to 2 drops lime essential oil
1 to 2 drops chamomile extract
Drops of water as needed

Instructions

1. Add honey, clay, and collagen to a small bowl. Mix the ingredients together.
2. Add lime essential oil and chamomile extract. Stir into the mix.
3. Stick your finger into the mix. If it's a consistency you like it's ready to apply to your skin. If not, add a few drops of water. Too much water will make your mix runny so use just a drop or two!
4. Apply the clay mask to your face and neck. Enhance your mix by adding additional extracts and essentials based on your needs. If you have sensitive skin, consider adding cucumber extract to the clay mix.
5. Keep this mix in the fridge and store for up to 10 days.

Chapter 8

Whipped, Buttered, and Creamed: How to Make the Best Hair and Body Butters

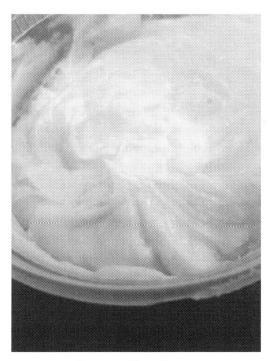

Coconut Shea Butter

Coconut Shea Butter

Coconut shea butter is soft and silky and will leave your skin indulgently moisturized and glowing. If you love using shea butter in your hair and haven't combined these two, stop what you're doing, go get the ingredients, and start making it now!

Ingredients

3 tablespoons raw, unrefined shea butter
2 tablespoons unrefined, organic coconut oil

Instructions

1. Stir coconut oil into your shea butter until well blended.
2. If your butters and oils are more firm, add them to your blender or mixing bowl.
3. Whip the ingredients until smooth, about 1 to 2 minutes.

This recipe makes a little under 4 ounces.

Optional: Add essential oils, two to four drops of your favorite. Vanilla essential oil goes well in this recipe.

Ingredient Benefits

You don't have to buy organic products to make wonderful natural goods. I've made many things with what I could afford, what was on sale, and what was actually working for me.

Since our skin is our largest organ, and whatever you put on it goes directly into your system, organic foods and products tend to have fewer toxins and pesticides. Those rules don't just apply to your edible products. Keep those pesticides out of your hair products too! Make sure to check those labels though. Make sure they are certified organic. As you know, not everything marked natural and organic isn't.

Coconut Oil Benefits

Coconut oil is packed with vitamin E, which makes it a wonderful moisturizer for your hair and skin.

There's a long list of coconut oil benefits, including:

- reduces frizz
- works as a natural emollient
- great deep conditioner
- a conditioning moisturizer for hair and skin
- gentle enough to be used on baby's skin (and their cute bottoms)
- adds natural shine to hair
- natural teeth whitener
- hair and skin softener
- helps hair retain moisture
- can be used as a lip and body scrub when combined with sugar

If you like to cook it up in the kitchen, coconut oil can be used as a tasty replacement for real butter. For a scrumptious recipe with coconut oil, check out my homemade butter recipe, Lavishly Butter in chapter 3. This butter is so good you won't go back to that other stuff. I promise.

Shea Butter Benefits

Shea butter is rich in vitamins A, E, D, essential fatty acids and allatonin (a product of uric acid that promotes the healing of skin wounds and infections). It's a little heavier than a lot of butters, so I like to combine it with lighter oils (safflower, sunflower) and butters.

Healing Effects

Shea butter has been used for chemo-prevention because of its many antitumor promoting effects. One study done in 2010 proved its anti-inflammatory and analgesic effects, specifically in the treatment of severe dermatitis.

Slick and Smooth

In addition to your body, use shea butter to seal in moisture after a wash and for styles that need a slick look. I like to use it to keep frizz away on ponytail days.

Green Tea Body Butter

Ingredients

1/4 cup avocado butter (melted)
1 teaspoon chia seed oil
1/2 teaspoon shea nut oil
1/8 teaspoon calendula extract
1/8 teaspoon green tea extract
6 to 8 drops of bergamot, sandalwood, or palmarosa essential oil

Instructions

1. Add oils and extracts to melted butters.
2. Stir and allow to cool for up to 8 hours.
3. You may also chill this fruit and veggie butter in the refrigerator for about 2 hours.

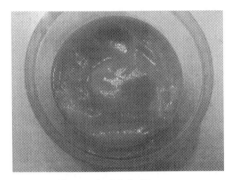

Organic Hair Butter

Organic Hair Butter

Ingredients

1 tablespoon organic shea butter
1/2 tablespoon organic coconut oil
1/2 tablespoon organic olive oil

Instructions

1. Simply melt the ingredients down in a heat-safe container or in a small pot on the lowest heat setting.
2. Remove from heat and let cool for 10 minutes.
3. Pour into a sealable jar.
4. Place in your refrigerator for up to 20 minutes, or in your freezer for 10 minutes.

Additional Options:

Add any (or all) of these options for a light, all-natural butter:

- 2 to 4 drops palmarosa essential oil
- 1 teaspoon aloe vera gel
- 1/2 tablespoon organic cocoa butter

Notes

This organic hair butter recipe won't weigh your hair down, provides your curls with deep moisture, eliminates frizz, and can be ready to use within a few minutes. My kind of hair butter!

This recipe makes about 2 ounces. If you need more, it's super simple to double. It's also a great moisturizer for hands, feet, and twinkly toes. Your butter will be firm but soft to the touch. It should easily melt on your fingers and into your hair.

Puff Butter

Ingredients

1/2 cup shea butter
1/4 cup cocoa butter
2 cups water
1/4 cup coconut oil

Instructions

1. Slowly heat your shea butter, cocoa butter and coconut oil in a heat-safe container that can sit in very hot water.
2. Bring 2 cups of water to a boil. Take the boiling water off of the heat. Let it cool for about 2 minutes,
3. Set your glass jar full of butters and oil inside the water. Stir occasionally to make sure everything is melting together.
4. Once everything has melted, allow the butter to cool. You can also place the butter in your refrigerator for up to 30 minutes, or until it is firm.

Quick Tip:

Add this butter to your mixer and whip it up for a different texture!!

This twist butter smells good enough to eat, and it only has three ingredients! In addition to being a wonderful hair butter, it's also awesome for hands, elbows, knees, and toes!

Kukui Nut Mango Butter

Ingredients

1/4 cup mango butter (softened)
1/4 cup shea butter (softened)
2 tablespoons kukui nut oil

Instructions

1. Combine all ingredients in a small pot if you're heating the ingredients on the stove.
2. Heat until the butter(s) and oils are soft enough to stir.
3. Let cool for about 10 to 15 minutes or until it can be poured in your airtight container.

Recipe Note

If your butters melt completely, place this butter in the freezer for about 15 minutes. Don't worry about the butter freezing into a hard piece of cement. It will still be nice and solid at room temperature. This butter will melt into your skin, hair, and fingertips while applying.

Twist and Braid Butter

Ingredients

2 tablespoons shea butter
1 tablespoon olive oil
6 drops orange essential oil
6 drops sandalwood essential oil

Instructions

1. Add the shea butter and olive oil to a sealable container.
2. Stir your ingredients.
3. Add in essential oils and stir.
4. Style and be fabulous!

Variation | Orange Sandalwood Twist and Braid Butter

Ingredients

2 tablespoons shea butter
1 tablespoon olive oil
6 drops orange essential oil
6 drops sandalwood essential oil
*optional: 3 drops lavender essential oil

Instructions

1. Add the shea butter and olive oil to a sealable container.
2. Stir your ingredients to desired consistency.
3. Add essential oils and stir.
4. Style and be fabulous!

Ingredient Spotlight

Shea Butter Benefits

One of the best things about shea butter is it's abiity to help replenish dull skin and a dry scalp. Shea butter is the luscious fat that is extracted from the nut (kernels) of the shea tree. It is the HBIC (head butter in charge) for most skin and hair regimens. It's health benefits are also pretty special. Current research suggests shea butter may help slow the growth of tumors and prevent cancer.[2] Researchers found shea butter to be:

1. Chemopreventive (to reduce the risk of, repress, suppress, reverse, or slow the development of cancer)[61]
2. Antimycobacterial (mycobacterial pathogens that cause diseases; examples: tuberculosis, leprosy)

Another study found that shea butter boosts production of collagen, which slows aging of the mind and body.[38] It also speeds the healing of wounds, rashes, skin irritations, and scars. Shea butter is wonderful to use on swollen feet or sore joints because it reduces inflammation.

It's extremely rich in:[2]

- Vitamin A - *great for the overall health and beauty of skin, hair*
- Vitamin E - *moisturizes and helps prevent hair loss*
- Vitamin F - *essential fatty acids; nourishes hair follicles; hair strengthener; prevents breakage; increases hair volume and thickness; heals, soothes, and hydrates hair and skin*

Olive Oil Benefits

Olive oil is easy to find and great for use in homemade hair and skin products.

Olive oil:

- *is good for the heart and decreases your risk of heart disease[67]*
- *contains vitamin E, great for hair and skin*
- *helps reduce inflammation in the body*
- *is packed with polyphenols and slows the growth of unwanted bacteria in the digestive tract, which helps decrease infection and lowers the risk of cancer in the digestive system[11]*
- *strengthens your bones*
- *improves cognition (memory, mental focus, and verbal fluency)*
- *promote healthy hair growth*
- *is a natural hair conditioner*
- *promotes hair shine*
- *is antimicrobial and antibacterial, which helps keep bacteria and fungus from growing on your scalp*
- *is a natural emollient that soothes and adds softness to hair and skin*

Orange Essential Oil

This lively fragrance has a naturally calming effect on your nervous system and boosts feelings of peace. It's even used to add flavor to beverages, desserts, and chocolate!

Orange essential oil (OE) is anti-inflammatory, a natural antidepressant, and an antiseptic oil. It is cold-pressed from the peels of oranges and is great for balancing oily skin. It's also wonderful in relieving itchy, dry scalp.

Orange essential oil is one of the safe essentials for use in homemade products for kids. The entire orange family promotes uplifting, cheerful thoughts and feelings. This applies to all orange scents, so experiment with tangerine, mandarin orange, or blood orange essential oils.

Sandalwood Essential Oil

Sandalwood is by far one of my favorite scents. I love it in hair butters because the scent lightly lingers without being overpowering and annoying. It's also an emollient and memory booster and is used in everything from medicines to deodorant!

Sandalwood is a natural astringent that helps tighten the skin and strengthens the muscles and gums (which is why you may find it in breath fresheners). It also soothes skin and helps heal scars. This centering fragrance boosts feelings of calmness, increases your ability to concentrate, and helps you stay in a good mood. It also helps reduce fear, anxiety, restlessness, and stress.

Whipped Apricot Shea Butter

Ingredients

1 cup shea butter
1 tablespoon apricot kernel oil
1 tablespoon olive oil
1/4 teaspoon aloe vera extract
10 drops lemon essential oil (or your favorite essential oil)
a glass jar with a lid

Instructions

This mix can be done by hand in a mixing bowl, or you can add ingredients to your blender or mixer. If you find your raw shea butter too hard to work with, heat 1 cup of water on medium-high for about 5 minutes. You can also warm some water in the microwave until it's almost boiling.

1. Place your shea butter in a heat-safe container or glass.
2. Set the cup in hot water. This will melt your shea butter gently while keeping all of its nutrient properties in place.
3. Pour in apricot kernel oil and olive oil.
4. Place your mixer on high and whip it!
5. Mix for about 2 minutes, then add aloe vera extract and lemon essential oil.
6. Blend on high speed for another minute. Transfer whipped shea butter into sealable jar or container.

Notes

Coconut oil is excellent in this mix. This recipe is flexible and will work well with 1 cup of raw, organic butter (shea, mango, cocoa, kokum, etc.) and 1/4 cup of your favorite oil.

Velvet

Velvet is made with all-natural, organic butters and oils you can find in most grocery stores. I'm using the coconut oil I buy from Trader Joe's in this recipe, but any coconut oil will work.

Ingredients

2 tablespoons cocoa butter
2 tablespoons shea butter
1/4 cup coconut oil
1 tablespoon avocado oil

Instructions

1. Gently melt all ingredients on the warm or low setting on top of the stove (or in your crockpot).
2. Warm for 5 minutes or until all ingredients have melted. Pour into a glass jar or heat-safe container to cool.
3. Allow the butter to cool for up to 4 hours, or place in the refrigerator for 30 minutes. Speed up the process by putting the butter in the freezer for about 10 minutes!

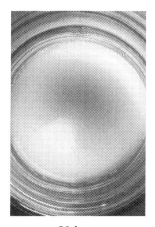

Velvet

Chapter 9

DIY Hair Oils, Infusions, & Cocktails

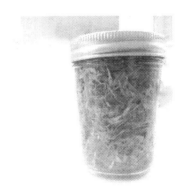

Calendula Oil

Ingredients

1 teaspoon fresh or dried rosemary
1 tablespoon fresh or dried lavender flowers
1/2 cup fresh or dried calendula flowers
4- to 6-ounce glass jar with lid
1/2 cup olive oil

Ingredients

1. Add flowers to your glass jar or airtight container. I use a 5-ounce jar for this recipe.
2. Gently press the flowers down into your jar so that you can add enough oil.
3. Add the oil.
4. Close the lid and let sit in one of your favorite windows for 6 to 8 weeks.

Don't have that long? Make this recipe in the crock pot!

Crockpot Instructions

1. Add the ingredients to your crockpot and use the warm or lowest setting.
2. Let the oil infuse for 20 to 30 minutes. Keep your eyes on it. Don't let your oil burn!
3. If making this on top of the stove, use the warm, simmer, or lowest setting and let it simmer for 30 to 45 minutes.
4. Once the oil is done, strain the flowers out and pour into a jar or container.

Note

Sunflower oil and safflower oil are great substitutions for olive oil in this recipe.

Captivating Calendula Flowers: Embrace the Power of the Marigold

Calendula oil (Calendula officials) is a light, moisturizing oil that adds shine and eliminates frizz. It's antimicrobial, antifungal, anti-inflammatory, and antiviral. It's also healing and soothing to the skin.[54] Cover these flowers with sunflower or olive oil and let it sit in a sunny window sill for up to eight weeks. You'll have a decadent oil that works well by itself and blends well with others!

Calendula oil comes from the petals of the marigold flower. These daisy-like flowers are often vibrant orange to bold yellow in color. This flower is most often used in aromatherapy to treat skin problems and wounds. It stimulates the production of collagen at the wound site, which helps reduce scarring. Calendula extract is a wonderful addition to add to your hair oil recipes. It prevents frizz, softens, smooths, and slicks edges for that perfect undo and adds extra shine.

Calendula Oil Benefits and Uses

- works as a natural emollient
- calms diaper rash and irritation
- reduces inflammation and pain[12]
- soothes and prevents chapped lips when used in lip balms
- great for sensitive skin
- soothes scalp irritation
- calendula tea can be used as a toner to heal acne
- reduces inflammation in skin conditions like eczema and dermatitis[12, 54]
- rejuvenating for hair and skin

How to Infuse Your Oils

When plants and essential oils get together, their healing potential increases more than if they were used alone. Infused oils are typically made by macerating or steeping plants, leaves, and roots in plant-based oils.[39] Herbs and plants can be used whole. You may also chop or grind dried herbs in your blender.

- Use a glass jar with a wide mouth and add your favorite flowers and oil.

- Keep the oil in a warm, dry place. Gently shake the oil daily, or at least three to four times a week.
- While infusing your oil, don't worry about fluctuations in temperature. Changes in the temperature will not damage the oil.
- Most oils are well infused after two weeks. The longer it infuses, the more color, aroma, and healing properties are released from the herbs and flowers. Let your nose be the judge!

To Ensure Herb Quality, Use Your Senses

There are a few things to keep in mind when shopping for dried herbs and flowers. What you see, smell, and taste matters! Make sure your botanicals are fresh and have the following three characteristics. They should be:[41]

1. Fragrant
2. Colorful
3. Organically grown or freshly picked (your backyard or inside garden is a great source)

Notes

Add fresh, dried lavender and rosemary leaves to the calendula oil. This will not only add natural fragrance but also boost feelings of relaxation and stimulate hair growth.

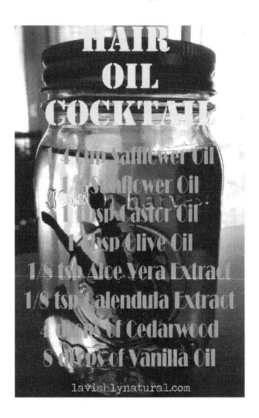

Lavishly Natural's Hair Oil Cocktail

Ingredients

1/4 cup sunflower oil
1 tablespoon castor oil
1 tablespoon olive oil
1/8 teaspoon green tea extract
1/8 teaspoon calendula extract
4 drops atlas cedarwood essential oil
8 drops vanilla essential oil
sealable plastic bottle or glass jar
optional: 2 tablespoons of dried lavender, pink or red roses, or calendula
flowers; 2 whole vanilla beans.

Instructions

1. Pour sunflower, castor, and olive oils into plastic bottle or glass jar. Stir in green tea extract, calendula extract and essential oils.
2. You may always infuse dried flowers and herbs into your oil. For a lavish option, add dried lavender, roses (pink or red), or calendula flowers.
3. This oil does not need to be heated. (It may be warmed for hot oil treatments and scalp massage.)
4. Infuse this cocktail for 2 weeks or up to 2 months with real vanilla beans.
5. Optional, slice the vanilla bean open and scoop out the seeds. Discard the vanilla pods. Vanilla oil can be pricey, but homemade. Wait for it … priceless! It will definitely make it a richer, more succulent oil for your curls.

Ingredient Spotlight

Safflower Oil (Botanical Name: Carthamus tinctorius)

It softens hair and skin. It's a medium to lightweight oil that's great to blend with sunflower oil. Wonderful alternative to nut oils for any allergy-sensitive naturalistas. We have nut allergies in our home and do not use almond oil, which is very popular (and awesome) and works well in this recipe.

Castor Oil (Botanical Name: Ricinus communis)

In the Middle Ages, the leaves of the castor bean plant were referred to as Palma Christi, the Palm of Christ.[48] This was due to its dynamic healing effects and curative abilities. Castor oil is described as a natural emollient that penetrates the skin easily. This thick, rich oil improves hair shine and overall greatness, seals moisture into hair strands and ends, and helps thicken and grow hair.

If the field of energy medicine could be represented in oil form, it would be castor oil!

Healing benefits of castor oil include:

- increases lymphatic circulation[60]
- relieves pain
- increases relaxation
- reduces nausea
- vibrational oil that brings physiological, emotional, mental, and spiritual balance[48]
- natural skin conditioner
- stimulates the liver
- antimicrobial[72]
- improves digestion

Its leaves, roots, and seed oil have been used to reduce inflammation, treat hypoglycemia and liver conditions, and as a natural laxative. Castor oil's antimicrobial effects are as strong as the antibiotic. In a recent study, castor oil was found to be as effective as ampicillin in treating chronic bacterial and staph infections.[48] Many naturalistas swear by its ability to thicken, grow, and increase the overall volume of natural hair.

Sunflower Oil (Botanical Name: Helianthus annuus)

An all-purpose carrier oil, sunflower is a light, sweet, greaseless oil that is packed with omega-6 and omega-9 essential fatty acids. It softens and smooths the skin[56] and is the perfect oil to use as a base for most massage oils. Blends well with other oils. Shelf life: twelve months.

Olive Oil (Botanical Name: Olea europaea, cold pressed)

Olive oil adds moisture to the scalp, making hair shinier and softer. Olive oil has antifungal and antibacterial properties. Its texture is heavy and oily … good to add to conditioner (1 tablespoon will work in any conditioner). Shelf life: one to two years.

Aloe Vera Extract (Botanical Name: Aloe barbadensis)

Excellent relief for dry hair, aloe vera extract is as awesome as her soul mates—aloe vera gel, the aloe plant, and the whole aloe family. Known to prevent hair loss and add moisture, and healing to damaged scalp and hair, aloe vera extract is a very light oil that adds extra lusciousness to your curls, kinks, and coils.

Calendula Extract (Botanical Name: Calendula officinalis)

Calendula extract helps relieve inflammation and lymphatic congestion. This helps speed the healing of wounds, bites, rashes, and skin irritations. It helps balance oily complexions and an oily scalp. It shuts down frizz and helps calm a busy mind. Add 1/8 teaspoon to your hair oils and leave-in conditioners. It eliminates frizz and adds softness and extra fabulousness to hair.

Cedarwood, Atlas (Botanical Name: Cedrus atlantica)

Warm, rich, and woodsy, this scent is excellent for any DIY recipes for that special person in your life (and not just because it's a natural aphrodisiac). Sexy cedarwood provides powerful stress relief (more than lavender), promotes hair growth, and helps prevent and clear the scalp of dandruff.

Vanilla Essential Oil (Botanical Name: Vanilla planifolia)

Vanilla is a magical member of the orchid family, which is one of the largest plant species on the planet. There's a growing body of research that shows vanillin, "a major component of vanilla[32]," prevents the spread of cancer and kills cancer cells.[50]

When added to your natural hair-care recipes, vanilla oil softens hair, heals the scalp, and helps you feel awesome! Science has found vanilla oil to have mood-boosting qualities that help you feel balanced and uplifted. It also works as a natural stress reliever, antidepressant, and libido enhancer.

Massage a little vanilla oil into your skin before bed. It will help you fall asleep faster and encourages good dreams.

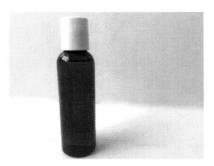

Homemade Vanilla Oil

Homemade Vanilla Oil

I often get asked what my absolute favorite recipe is, or the one I can't live without. If I had to pick just one thing, it would be this—homemade vanilla oil.

Why?

It's luxurious, tells frizz to have several seats, is excellent for skin, and gets even better over time. Did you know vanilla oil has some crazy medicinal properties?

Vanilla oil:

- relieves nausea
- lowers blood pressure
- may reduce the percentage of sickled cells in individuals with sickled cell anemia
- is a natural sedative that induces sleep
- has antidepressant properties that lift mood, dissolve anger, and promote good feelings
- soothes all types of inflammation and hyperactivity in the mind and body

- helps regulate menstruation
- alleviates insomnia
- improves sexual function, behavior, and arousal

Ingredients

1 cup safflower oil
1/2 cup apricot kernel oil
1/2 cup sunflower oil
1/4 cup cocoa butter (melted)
4 to 6 whole, ground, or cut vanilla beans

Instructions

1. Add ingredients to glass jar.
2. Let the oil sit in the sun for up to 8 weeks.
3. Strain the vanilla beans from your oil and enjoy!
4. This oil has a shelf life of 1 to 2 years.

Ridiculous Recipe Extras

Erica's Buttery Vanilla Oil Recipe

This is a basic vanilla oil recipe that gets better with time. Place the following ingredients in a festive purple or green jar and let sit in a warm, dry place or on a sunny windowsill for a minimum of 8 weeks. Strain the vanilla beans. Store in a 16-ounce jar or bottle.

Ingredients

2 cups safflower oil (or sunflower oil)
1/4 cocoa butter (melted)
4 to 6 whole, cut, or sliced vanilla beans

Additional Ways to Make Vanilla Oil

Crockpot Recipe

Add safflower oil, whole vanilla beans, and cocoa butter to crockpot. Use the warm setting for about 30 minutes. Turn off the heat and add 10 drops of vanilla essential oil.

(Do not bring oil to a boil.)

Stovetop Recipe

Put all the ingredients in a quart-sized pot. Turn the stove to the lowest setting and let it simmer for up to an hour. Lavish it up with hair-loving dried botanicals like pink or red roses, lavender, hibiscus, or chamomile flowers. All four are wonderful for your hair and skin.

Vanilla Mint Hair Repair Oil

Ingredients

1/4 cup safflower oil
1/4 cup apricot kernel oil
1 tablespoon coconut oil (liquid)
1 tablespoon avocado oil
4 drops rose hip seed oil
1/4 teaspoon vitamin E
6 drops vanilla essential oil
2 drops peppermint essential oil

Instructions

1. Combine safflower, apricot kernel, coconut and avocado oils in a bottle or container.
2. Add rose hip seed oil.
3. Add vitamin E and vanilla and peppermint essential oils.

Great for use as a hot oil treatment, scalp and hair nourishment, scalp massage, hair repair, replenishment shine. And it smells like Christmas! It's also wonderful after a shower and when added to a bath.

Homemade Carrot Cake Oil

Ingredients

2 carrots
2 whole vanilla beans
2 cups safflower oil
1 teaspoon vitamin e
16 ounce bottle

Instructions

1. Wash and peel your carrots.
2. Grate and add them to your crockpot.
3. Gently cut open your vanilla bean with a knife. Scoop out the vanilla beans and add them to the crockpot. Add the empty vanilla pod and your oils.
4. Put your crockpot on the warm setting. Warm the oil on the lowest heat setting for up to an hour. You don't want your it to burn or get to hot. It should not be smoking!
5. Strain the carrots and goodies from the oil and discard.
6. Pour the oil into your bottle and it's good to go! Use this as a finishing oil, to help seal your ends, after shower oil, or skin moisturizer.

I let the carrot oil simmer on the warm setting for about 2 hours and then let it cool overnight. As soon as the oil cools, add in the Vitamin E.

Notes

This oil is great to use for hot oil treatments, styling, facial serums, and scalp massage. I like to add 3 or 4 whole vanilla beans to this recipe, I can't have too much! This gives your oil a beautiful carrot cake smell!

The Healing Oil

1/2 cup organic sunflower oil
1/2 cup organic safflower oil
1/4 cup avocado oil
15 drops sandalwood essential oil
10 drops rose essential oil

Instructions

1. Pour safflower and avocado oil into an 16 ounce (2 cups) squeeze bottle. Gently shake the bottle to blend oils.
2. Add in essential oils and shake for a few about 30 seconds.
3. If using this blend for infant massage or with little children, try blending 2 drops of vanilla essential oil or orange essential oil instead of sandalwood and rose.

Ingredient Spotlight

Safflower Oil (Conditioning)

Safflower oil, when added to my clay washes, hot oil treatments, and cosmetics, gives my hair shine that can be seen without squinting! It conditions the skin, is high in unsaturated fatty acids that strengthen the hair, and gives your body a radiant, healthy glow!

Apricot Kernel Oil (Restoring)

This oil is a perfect substitute for almond oil in that its consistency and function are similar. Since I'm a naturalista with nut allergies, I stumbled across this oil when looking for non-greasy, nut-free oils for hair and skin.

Apricot oil absorbs quickly, leaving a silky feel. This makes it perfect for use as a massage oil, as well as in soaps and cosmetics. It's high in essential fatty acids (omega-3, 6, and 9) and gives the benefits of a rich, thick oil without the oily-ness. Plus, if you're using it as a massage oil, it won't leave your sheets oily or sticky.

Coconut Oil (Healing)

Coconut oil is a powerful emollient that smooths and heals the skin. It has anti-inflammatory benefits and is antibacterial and deeply moisturizing. When used as part of your pre- or post-wash regime, coconut oil prevents protein loss from the hair shaft (in damaged and undamaged hair).[41] This gives you stronger, healthier hair and prevents split ends.

Coconut oil:

- *reverses thinning hair*
- *helps hair retain moisture, preventing breakage*
- *makes a powerful conditioner by itself, when warmed before applying to your hair*
- *keeps hair soft and supple*
- *can reduce the appearance of split ends and heal them*
- *prevents baldness and gray hair*

Avocado Oil (nourishing)

Avocado oil is rich in Vitamin A and essential and trace minerals, which are great for preventing hair loss. It is also used to treat the thickening of the skin (sclerosis) and gum infections. Since it soothes and heals the skin so well and stimulates blood flow to the scalp, it promotes hair growth and speeds wound healing. Add 1 teaspoon of avocado oil to your favorite conditioner for a lavish conditioning experience!

Rosehip Seed Oil (rejuvenating)

Rosehip seed oil is high in omega-3, omega-6, and omega-9 essential fatty acids. These are great for healing the skin, improving brain function, and balancing our mood. This oil is excellent for repairing damage to the skin and for skin rejuvenation. It's also effective as a natural moisturizer for sensitive skin.

Peppermint Essential Oil (revitalizing)

Peppermint oil has ancient roots as a medicinal oil. My love of peppermint and peppermint oil runs deep, and that's a good thing because it's a powerful healing herb that's awesome for hair growth! If you ever eat a little too much or something that doesn't agree with your greatness, get rid of that upset stomach with hot peppermint tea. It stops nausea in its tracks!

Peppermint oil benefits:

- o   stimulates blood flow to the scalp
- o   promotes healthy hair growth
- o   used to treat irritable bowel syndrome
- o   prevents dry, cracked nipples while breastfeeding

Vanilla essential oil (calming) benefits:

- •   reduces stress
- •   calms the mind
- •   helps regulate menstruation[63]
- •   reduces nausea

Cedar wood Essential Oil (Stimulating)

Cedarwood essential oil is stimulating to the scalp. It is often used as an all-natural cleanser. A few drops added to your daily spritz, or gently massaged into your scalp for a pre-poo, is all that's needed to begin seeing the benefits. It has antiseptic, astringent and healing properties that relieve itching and reduce skin eruptions.[40]

Cedarwood essential oil is anti-seborrhoeic (seborrhea or eczema). This means that it prevents and balances excess secretions from the sebaceous glands. This is important when treating conditions like eczema.

Eczema occurs when there is a malfunctioning of sebaceous glands, which increases sebum production and infection of the epidermal cells. Cedarwood helps reduce the skin peeling and inflammation that can come with this condition.

Next time you're having a muscle spasm, try massaging some cedarwood into the area (mix it with a tablespoon of olive oil). It's antispasmodic, meaning it relieves muscle spasms and spasms of the heart, intestines, respiratory system, and nerves.

Other health benefits of cedarwood:

- cures acne
- acts as an all-natural mosquito repellant
- improves the quality of sleep, works well as a sedative[41]
- stimulates metabolism
- regulates menstruation

Ylang Ylang Essential Oil (Balancing)

This essential oil balances the natural sebum in your scalp, prevents hair loss, and stimulates hair growth. Ylang ylang has many health benefits, including:

- helps lower blood pressure
- decreases the symptoms of depression
- effective for sensitive, oily, or acne-prone skin
- a powerful hair tonic when blended with any carrier oil (especially jojoba)
- balances oil production in all skin types

- strengthens your intuition
- decreases feelings of anger, frustration, fear, and jealousy

Sage Essential Oil (Strengthening)

Sage essential oil was once used to preserve food due to its powerful antioxidant properties. It's earlier medicinal uses were for the reduction of epilepsy and neurodevelopmental conditions. Sage is now used as a decongestant and to relieve infections of the throat and mouth.

Here are some other health benefits of sage oil:

- natural scalp and hair tonic, antifungal, antimicrobial, antibacterial, anti-inflammatory
- restores alertness
- induces mental stability
- is estrogenic, meaning it influences hormonal action in the form of "regulating the menstrual cycle, decreasing lactation, and alleviating menopause symptoms."[31]
- helps prevent hair loss
- increases the flow of creative ideas

Sage essential oil should not be used during pregnancy.

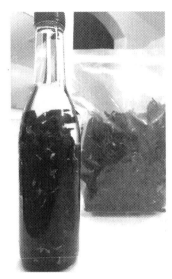

Organic Hibiscus Hair Oil

Organic Hibiscus Hair Oil

This is a light, luscious oil that adds softness and sheen to your hair. A naturalista favorite for hair growth, this oil is perfect for detangling, hot oil treatments, twists, braids, and oil rinsing!

Milady's Skin Care and Cosmetics Ingredients Dictionary[74] didn't have a description of hibiscus oil, but it did have some things to say about hibiscus extract:

- It's moisturizing and refreshing.
- It provides a tightening effect without stripping the skin of its natural oils.
- It is recommended for oily skin due to its high degree of astringency and its toning properties.
- The extract is obtained from the flowers.
- There are over two hundred varieties of this plant.

Organic Hibiscus Hair Oil Recipe

Ingredients

1 cup organic sunflower oil
1/2 cup organic coconut oil
1/2 cup organic hibiscus flowers

Instructions

1. Add ingredients to quart-sized pot.
2. Bring to a boil, then turn off heat.
3. Let the oil completely cool in the pot for about 15 minutes.
4. Strain the hibiscus flower from the oil and discard.
5. Pour hibiscus oil into 12-ounce bottle or jar and enjoy!

Sun Goddess | Infused Oil Recipe

Ingredients

1/2 cup organic sunflower oil
1/2 cup safflower oil
1/2 cup organic coconut oil
1/2 cup organic hibiscus flowers
handful of dried lavender, calendula, roses, or chamomile flowers

Instructions

1. Add all the ingredients to a sealable glass jar or container.
2. Seal jar and place in a sunny window (direct or indirect light) for up to 8 weeks.
3. Optional: 6 drops of palmarosa essential oil for fragrance.

Lavishly Lavender Oil

Lavender oil is great for calming your nerves, repelling scorpians, mosquitos and even healing itchy mosquito bites! It's also one of the best oils your can use to prevent hair loss and alopecia.[44]

Ingredients

1/2 cup dried lavender buds
1 cup safflower oil
1 teaspoon Vitamin E
8 ounce glass jar with lid

Instructions

1. Place dried lavender flowers, leaves and buds to glass jar.
2. Pour oil over the flowers. Make sure all of the flowers are covered.
3. Allow this oil to sit in a place that gets lots of natural light for 2 months (any happy window sill will work:).
4. Once a week, shake the oil and return it to it's sunny place.
5. After 2 months, open the oil and strain out all of the flower buds. Throw the flower buds away.
6. Pour the oil into a glass jar and add the Vitamin E. Stir or gently shake the oil and it's ready for use! Store this oil in a cool, dry place. It will stay fresh for up to 6 months.

Recipe Note

Lavishly Lavender: How To Make Homemade Lavender Oil
LavishlyNatural.com/Lavenderoil

Relax Goddess After Bath Oil

2 cups water
3/4 cup sunflower oil
1/4 cup apricot oil
8 to 10 drops of any one of the following essential oils: lavender, rosewood, sage, or holy basil

Instructions

1. Boil 2 cups of water and remove from heat.
2. Measure your oils and place them in a heat-safe container.
3. Place the container in the hot water and let it sit for 5 minutes or until your oil is warm.
4. Pour half the oil in your bottle.
5. Add essential oils and gently shake the bottle.
6. Add remaining oil. You're good to go!

Ingredient Benefits

Apricot Oil (Also known as apricot kernel oil.)

Rich with vitamins A, E, and C, this nourishing oil deeply moisturizes the skin. The oil comes from the apricot kernel of the apricot pit. It's lightweight, nongreasy, and absorbs directly into the skin. It leaves the skin feeling silky and smooth.

Its anti-inflammatory properties allow it to be soothing for all skin types. It's a soothing oil for skin conditions like eczema and dermatitis. It's also very high in gamma linoleic acids, which allows skin to maintain its natural moisture balance. Apricot oil's lubricating nature makes it wonderful for massage, and it won't mess up your sheets.

Safflower Oil

Considered to be a dry oil, safflower oil doesn't leave your skin feeling oily. This may be one of the reasons it's considered a wonderful carrier oil for massage blends. It's high in omega-6 fatty acids (linoleic acid), which help keep the skin impermeable to water.

Safflower oil is soothing to the mind and body. It helps relieve poor circulation in the legs, reduces the inflammation of swollen feet, and prevents dandruff and hair breakage. Safflower oil absorbs easily into the skin and combines well with other oilier oils like avocado, olive, jojoba, and apricot.

Any one of the following essential oils are suggested:

Ylang Ylang Essential Oil (EO)

Stronger scent; sweet, floral; works as a sedative, so use in low amounts; natural aphrodisiac; makes your senses more alert; dissolves negative energy.

Rosewood EO

Sweet, rosy and woodsy fragrance; helps rejuvenate the cells; encourages tranquility and eases headaches; increases feelings of sensuality and peace; improves communication.

Sandalwood EO

Soft, warm, and woodsy; promotes peaceful relaxation and openness; balances giving and receiving energy; raises vibration of abundance and prosperity.

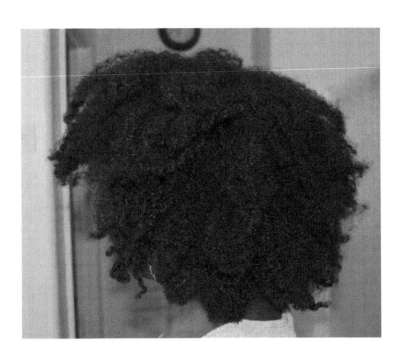

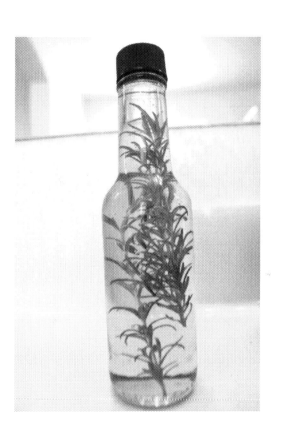

Chapter 10

How To Make Your Own Mega Hair-Growth Serum

This recipe uses all natural plant oils, essential oils that speed hair growth, and castor oil that prevents and speeds the healing of wounds and skin irritation. Since you've just completed your ingredient list and you know what your hair enjoys, consider using a carrier oil that you know your hair loves. A carrier oil is usually a plant-based oil that's used to dilute essential oils.

You can use any essential oils that you saw repeated in the products you buy most often. Most essential oils like ylang ylang, or the citrus oils (lemon, orange, tangerine, lime) are affordable and packed with healthy hair and skin benefits. In the next section, we'll explore some essential oils that are perfect for any hair recipe.

If you're not sure which products or ingredients to use, no worries! Each ingredient in this serum has some serious hair-growth powers. Read about each of them in the benefits section below.

Here's the basic recipe:

1/8 teaspoon of essential oil (or 60 drops)
4 tablespoons of carrier oil (2 ounces)

The oils I'll be using are:

- organic safflower oil (carrier oil)
- castor oil
- rosemary essential oil
- basil essential oil
- cedarwood essential oil

Mega Hair-Growth Serum

A simply serum that also reduces hair shedding, adds shine, and stimulates hair growth.

Ingredients

2 tablespoons safflower oil
10 drops rosemary essential oil
10 drops basil essential oil
10 drops cedarwood essential oil
2 tablespoons castor oil

Instructions

1. Pour safflower oil into jar.
2. Add essential oils.
3. Add castor oil.
4. Shake, shake, shake—and apply!

Optional:

Add 1/8 teaspoon of calendula oil for silkiness; add two drops of broccoli seed extract for healthy scalp and to boost hair growth.

Mega Hair-Growth Serum Benefits

The Carrier | Safflower Oil

Safflower oil is described by *Milady's Skin Care and Cosmetics Ingredients Dictionary* (2010) as a carrier oil that is "hydrating to the skin" (p. 268). Safflower oil is a light, fragrance-free oil that is high in essential fatty acids and triglycerides. These nutrients are excellent for:

- *increasing circulation to the scalp*
- *stimulating hair growth*
- *strengthening hair follicles*
- *keeping hair shiny and vibrant*

Safflower oil has some of the highest nutrients of all carrier oils and blends very well with other essential oils.

Essentials Oils For Mega Hair Growth

The Boss | Rosemary Essential Oil

This oil has so many benefits I couldn't begin to list them all … but I tried!

Twenty-One Benefits of Rosemary Essential Oil

1. Stimulates hair growth
2. Beneficial for acne, dermatitis, and eczema
3. Improves poor circulation
4. An ancient remedy for dandruff and hair loss
5. Helps eliminate cellulite
6. Detoxifies the liver
7. Often used for masking odor and providing fragrance in cosmetics[41]
8. Lowers cholesterol
9. Natural stress reliever
10. Eases muscle and rheumatism pain

11. Calms the digestive system
12. Relieves bloating
13. Treats lung congestion, sore throat, and canker sores
14. Stimulates the nervous system, motor nerves, adrenals, and a sluggish gallbladder
15. Improves memory
16. Helps increase concentration
17. Great remedy for forgetfulness, mental fatigue, and depression
18. Strengthens perception and creativity
19. Helps balance mind and body
20. Prevents dizziness
21. Helps you remember good dreams

The Motivator | Bodacious Basil Essential Oil

Milady's Skin Care and Cosmetics Ingredients Dictionary (2010) describes basil oil as "stimulating, purifying, and antimicrobial." (p. 103)

Big basil's benefits include:

- promotes hair growth
- relieves headaches, sinus congestion, and head colds
- treats nausea, shingles, herpes, indigestion, and sore muscles
- stimulates adrenals
- stimulates the production of breast milk
- helps balance oily skin
- has an uplifting effect
- confidence booster
- increases awareness

The Healer | Soothing Cedarwood Essential Oil

Cedarwood is a natural antiseptic that blends well with other oils. Its benefits include:

- fights hair loss
- relieves dandruff
- heals acne
- improves sleep quality
- stimulates circulation
- a natural astringent for oily and congested skin conditions
- soothes bug bites and itching
- clarifies and inspires the mind
- sedates nerves[40]

Recipe Extras | The 7 Essentials Oils You Can Use for Any Recipe

A question I get quite often on through my blog is:

"Which essential oil should I use for my hair?"

Sometimes the question is more specific or about a particular hair goal. My first recommendation is always the citrus oils. I love using them in almost every homemade recipe. Some that I keep in my home salon are: *lemon, tangerine, sweet orange, bergamot, lime, and grapefruit.*

All citrus oils have an uplifting energy. They boost mood and attract joy in some way. You just feel good when they're around! They're also more affordable than most other essentials (bergamot can get up there sometimes:). As much as I love the citrus oils, there are thousands to choose from and trying to figure out which ones are great for hair, can be a challenge.

The Best Essential Oils for Natural Hair, Mind & Body

In the next section I've included a list of the 7 Essentials that will give you the quickest results. If you want a recipe boost, blend your essentials.

Some examples:

If you're interested in stopping hair shedding and some inconvenient cramps, try a patuchouli and sweet orange blend.

Interested in boosting positive energy, lifting mood, or blessing yourself and the space you're in — add grapefruit, geranium or ylang ylang to your recipes.

Quick Tip

Place 4 to 6 drops of any of the essential oils that follow into 1/2 cup of distilled water. Pour it into a spray bottle and use it as a spritz to clear the energy in a room, and to give your gorgous skin a hydrating mist!

Ingredient Spotlight | The 7 Essentials

1. Grapefruit Essential Oil

Natural antidepressant; promotes positive feelings, hopefulness, and relaxation. Excellent overall health tonic for hair, mind, and body. Helps balance oily skin.

2. Clary Sage

Natural relaxant; antidepressant; reduces muscle spasms; natural aphrodisiac; heals rashes; reduces inflammation; induces feelings of euphoria, joy, and confidence; helpful in breaking addictions.

3. Geranium

Improves skin; reduces blood pressure; antibacterial; helps in the regeneration of new cells; uplifting; strengthens mental functioning.

4. Patchouli

Cell rejuvenator; antifungal; reduces appetite; conditions hair; eliminates dandruff; enhances sensuality; good for centering and meditation.

5. Rose Bulgarian

Decreases nervous tension; mind calming; boosts libido; improves memory; antibacterial; decreases nausea; improves circulation.

6. Sweet orange

Uplifting, cheerful, antidepressant; relieves cramps; boosts the immune system. This is my favorite essential for homemade hair and skin goodies for kids. Team Lavish refers to this scent as Fruit Snacks. We add it to baths, hair, and body oils.

7. Ylang Ylang

Anger eliminator; dissolves anxiety; helps reduce blood pressure; balancing/centering properties; clears negative thoughts; reduces dermatitis.

Chapter 11

Behavioral Nutrition: Edible Recipes For Hair Growth and Wellness

Purification and Rejuvenation as a way of life—A wonderful, fantastic, ecstatic fulfilling way of living. A gift supreme. Explosive! Oh so powerful! Makes you feel clean on the inside. Look beautiful on the outside. Embrace your healing, digest it, caress it, fall back on it, move forward with it, stand on it, lean on it, rest on it. It will build you into a perfect temple of pure light, love, wealth, and health.
—Queen Afua, Heal Thyself

Eat Your Hair-Growth Vitamins

By Morwena (Mo) Gould, Reiki Therapist, Self-Esteem Coach

You already understand that your body and luscious curls are made from the foods you eat. This section will help you understand exactly which foods are best to grow a magnificent mane from the inside out!

Learn the secrets of gluten-free living and understand the huge physical and mental benefits you can experience each time you add more gluten-free options to your diet. Are you ready to calm your mind and nourish your hair with the food-based secrets I have to share?

Food That's Alive!

When we pluck an apple from tree (or purchase one organically), it is still alive. The fresh colors, the smell, the juicy taste all mean it is still living. When the food "dies," changes occur to the color, taste, and texture. When apples die, they go brown and mushy!

When we cook foods, it has a similar impact. Brown, mushy cooked apples may taste delicious, but we have still killed the food. The changes in color and texture are the result of enzymes breaking down the food; this is part of the natural process. In the wild, plants are recycled back into organic matter in the soil to nourish future generations.

When foods are alive, they contain fresh enzymes that are beneficial for your body[4]; they help you digest the food. Alive, specifically uncooked foods contain beneficial vitamins and other biological compounds that are frequently destroyed by cooking. Raw and living food is more alive and, in many cases, more beneficial to your body.

There are some foods, like tomatoes, which when cooked have a greater amount of nutrients for your body to absorb, and some nutrients need to be eaten with fat to help you absorb them. Having a balance of cooked and fresh fruit and vegetables is essential to increasing your vitality and ensuring you get the spectrum of nutrition needed for you and your hair!

Follicular Engineering

Understanding how hair is produced by your body is vital to making nourishing decisions. Your hair grows from its root, which is called the follicle, a special bit of skin. This skin has its own blood supply and takes food from your blood to make the hair. The hair itself is made out of a rigid protein called keratin made from eighteen different amino acids (protein building blocks).

As your hair grows, it gets pushed up through the follicle and gets oiled along the way by a special gland that conditions the hair with your own magical oil. A sheath within the follicle surrounds the hair and protects it until it is ready to be revealed to the outside world!

In order to give your hair the best chance to grow optimally, you need to provide the correct nutrients!

From the table that follows, you can see how vitally important it is to consume plenty of fruits and vegetables to get all the healthy hair nutrients. Many of these nutrients work better and reach you in larger amounts when you get them from food in its raw and most natural state.

Once you understand which foods you can add to your diet to improve your hair and overall well-being, we'll have a quick look at some foods that you may like to consider quitting!

Nutrient	Why It Is Needed	Good Sources
Essential amino acids (specifically methionine and cysteine)	Provides building blocks for hair and follicles	High-quality proteins (nuts, seeds, grass-fed meat, wild salmon, avocado)
Antioxidants	Prevents DNA damage and promotes DNA repair	Raw fruit and vegetables (for example, a lovely juice!)
Biotin (water-soluble B vitamin)	Protects hair and prevents breakage	Almonds, liver, egg yolk, oats, brown rice, yeast
Omega-3 fatty acids	Needed for oil production and healthy skin, brain development and healthy function	Salmon, eggs, flax seed, walnuts

Beta-carotene (vitamin A precursor)	Used by the body to make vitamin A and encourages hair growth	Sweet potatoes, carrots, spinach, broccoli
Vitamin C	Strengthens follicle and prevents breakage by increasing collagen	Citrus fruits, yellow or red bell peppers, strawberries
Vitamin E	Enhances blood flow and speeds up hair growth, prevents breakages	Sunflower seeds, almonds, pine nuts, dried apricots, cooked spinach, and olives
Methylsulfonylmethane	Increases keratin production and strengthens follicles	Raw leafy vegetables (alfalfa, Swiss chard, cabbage and watercress) or cooked asparagus, beets
Glutathione	an antioxidant found in every cell; helps the body methylate and detox toxins from the cell; prevents cellular damage; helps the body recover	(all organic) broccoli, cauliflower, squash, garlic, onions, avocados, tomatoes
Iron	Essential for oxygen transport in the blood and hair growth, needs vitamin C for proper absorption	Green leafy vegetables, leeks, dried fruits, figs, and berries

Silica	Balances hormones that control hair growth phases	Cucumber, mango, kale, spinach, greens (collard, mustard), kidney beans, celery, asparagus
Iodine	Increase thyroid activity and improves scalp condition	Kelp, nori, dulse, kombu, and wakame
Zinc	Improves scalp condition, prevents hair loss	strawberries, chickpeas, oatmeal, pumpkin seeds, sweet potato, seseame seeds, cucumbers

What's Wrong With Bread?

Bread is not the same as it used to be. During the industrialization of bread, manufacturers made some significant changes that are dramatically impacting our health today:

- Removing the bran from the germ of the grain gives bread a longer shelf life, but it also removes a lot of nutrients.
- Adding twenty-five different chemicals, additives, bleaches, and preservatives strips almost all the natural vitamins and minerals and fills it with toxic chemicals that the body needs to process.[19]
- Fortifying and enriching the flour (since the previous processing step removed nutrients) confuses the body with synthetic vitamins and minerals made from industrial chemicals and ingredients. The confused body then attacks the synthetic nutrients and, most worryingly, itself too.
- Modern wheat has been engineered to be a high-yield, dwarf wheat that contains more protein-gluten and wheat germ agglutinin

(WGA), which acts like an opioid drug in the brain, making it more addictive.

Impact of Gluten

Bread tastes delicious because of the addictive nature of modern wheat; it's tricking your brain! It is also wreaking havoc on your body in a whole host of other ways. A gluten senstivity symptoms can be very wide, ranging from lethargy and bloating to dizziness and foggy thoughts.[55]

How do you feel after eating some bread?

Are you full of life and ready to rock, or do you need a three-hour nap? Let your body tell you how it feels about gluten and find out firsthand what you experience when you eat it.

One More Thing (from Erica)

Gluten can be found in the places you least expect. You may recognize many of the gluten sources on this list. The best way to tell if you are affected by gluten is to remove it from your diet, and see how you feel. Gluten-free is used to market products, so keep in mind, not everything that says "gluten-free" is. Check the labels and the ingredients to be sure.

My son doesn't have Celiac Disease, but he does have a severe gluten allergy. As part of his autism recovery, his doctor put him on a gluten-free diet over 4 years ago. It's helped improve his neurological function, cogntive development and speech. Even though we eat gluten-free, I've found gluten can sneak up in anything, even your lipstick!

The Celiac Disease Foundation (2017) has an extensive list on their website of many sources. Here is a brief list...

Sources of Gluten[13]

- **wheat and wheat variations:**
  durham
  farro
  seminola
  spelt
  wheatberries
  graham
- **rye**
- **barley**
- **brewer's yeast**
- malt (malted milk shakes, malt extract, malted milk, malt flour, and yes — beer)
- pastas
- noodles
- pastries
- cookies
- donuts
- granola
- croutons
- flour tortillas
- brown rice syrup
- french fries
- potato chips
- soy sauce
- salad dressings and marianades
- vitamins and supplements

Intolerant or Just Sensitive?

Gluten is made of two different proteins (glutelin and gliadin), and it gives bread its soft and chewy texture. Celiac disease is a condition where people develop severe allergies to gluten, and it is categorized as an autoimmune condition. Really this is just a sign that the body is in a state of panic, and the bowel damage caused by the autoimmunity reduces nutrient uptake.

Gluten sensitivity is a more modern condition with little or no gastrointestinal problems but is often associated with mental health issues. Needless to say, the medical and food conglomerates are not keen to recognize this alarming association!

It is believed that the proteins are not properly digested and instead turn into substances similar to opium and impact certain areas of the brain, reducing our natural balance of neurotransmitters and happy chemicals. Studies have clearly shown an improvement in the symptoms of many neuroloical and mental health conditions by removing gluten from the diet.[10]

Make Me! | A Kick-Awesome Gluten-Free Recipe

This recipe a new twist on an old favorite, onion rings! It has all of the elements of a perfect gluten free recipe — it's easy to make, not labor intensive, and they taste like the best onion rings you've had in a while! If you have little ones, they tend to love these and have no idea how healthy they are:)

The Kings Onion Rings

Ingredients

1 cup chickpea flour
2 tablespoons arrowroot powder
1 teaspoon baking powder
1 teaspoon salt
2/3 cup seltzer water
2 flaxseed eggs
2 onions
2 cups sunflower oil
strainer
spoon (wooden or heat-resistant)
a super sharp knife
a small pot with tall sides

Instructions

1. Add sunflower oil to your pot and turn it to low heat. Slice onions 1/2 inch thick.
2. In a medium bowl, add chickpea flour, arrowroot powder, baking powder and salt. Whisk the ingredients.
3. Add in flaxseed egg (directions at the bottom) and seltzer water to the dry ingredients. Whisk until everything is combined.
4. Turn the oil to medium-high heat. Place a handful of onions into the batter. Gently stir until all of the onions are coated with the batter.

5. Drop by the handful into the oil. Cook on each side for 4 to 6 mnutes, or until the onion rings turn a light brown color.
6. Remove from the oil with the heat reisistant spoon and place in your strainer.
7. Repeat this process with the rest of the batter. These are great by themselves or served with a wheat-free ketchup!

Note

If you don't have arrowroot powder, use cornstarch. It works the same way.

Fascinating Flaxseed Egg Recipe

- 1 tablespoon ground flaxseed
- 3 tablespoons hot water (can be boiling)

If you're making your own ground flaxseeds:

Grind 1/2 cup of whole flaxseeds in a high-speed blender for up to 30 seconds.

Flaxseed Egg Instructions

1. Whisk or stir flaxseeds, then let them sit for 8 to 10 minutes.
2. Whisk again incorporate any remaining water. Add the flaxseed egg to your recipe.

This butter will last in your refrigerator for up to 3 months.

Chapter 12

Natural Milk: Awesome Allergy-Free Options

Grab some chia seeds and raise a glass to these six seriously awesome dairy-free milk recipes!

Coconut Milk & Friends

If you can't tell by now, I put just about everything in my hair! I've used coconut milk, cream, and manna to make deeply conditioning hair treatments like henna and chocolate (page). It leaves hair soft, silky, and deeply moisturized. A great help when I'm wearing styles where I want to minimize frizz and keep detangling a tropical breeze!

More healthy hair benefits of coconut milk include:

- contains lauric acid, which is antifungal, antibacterial, and antiviral (no more funkiness in the scalp)
- high in fatty acids that replenish and rehydrate
- reduces split ends
- helps remove dirt and excess sebum from hair and skin
- adds natural shine
- packed with vitamin, E which is a natural hair and skin moisturizer

- nourishes hair
- prevents dandruff

Besides the high fiber and B vitamin content, coconut milk may aid the body's protection of viruses and infections. Coconuts contain lauric acid, a medium-chain saturated fatty acid that the body converts into monolaurin. This highly beneficial compound is an antiviral and antibacterial that destroys a wide range of disease-causing organisms.

Coconut milk is also packed with magnesium, phosphorous, iron, vitamin C, calcium, sodium, and selenium. The most delicious and wholesome milk or cream, it adds decadence and coconut flavor to any meal. It is packed full of vitamins and minerals and has a naturally sweet taste.

How To Make Coconut Milk

Recipe Essentials:

High-speed blender
Medium-sized pot
Mesh strainer
1 gallon bottle with sealable top

Ingredients

1 cup coconut flakes
4 cups boilng water

Instructions

1. Pour the water into a 2-quart pot and bring to a boil.
2. While the water is heating, add coconut flakes to a high-speed blender.

3. Blend for up to 1 minute or until the flakes become a soft powder. You may have to stop your blender and wipe down the sides a few times to get a soft powder.

4. Remove boiling water from the heat and allow it to cool off for 5 minutes. Pour water into your high speed blender with the coconut powder. Allow the coconut powder to soften in the water for 2 to 3 minutes before you blend. This will help your milk blend faster and have more taste.

5. Blend on high for 4 minutes.

6. Pour the coconut milk through a strainer 2 o 3 times or until the milk pours through the strainer without leaving any pulp behind.

7. Pour your coconut milk into your bottle. It will store in your refrigerator for up to 3 weeks. Shake your coconut milk before drinking. If you it turns into a solid after leaving it in the refrigerator, allow it to sit out for a few minutes, shake and enjoy!

What To Do With That Leftover Coconut Pulp
A Quick Coconut Flour Recipe

1. If you have a dehydrator, save the coconut pulp you strain from your milk. Allow it to dry in your dehydrator on 110 degrees for up to 4 hours.

2. Once it dries, add it to your blender and blend until it becomes a fine powdery flour (2 to 4 minutes).

Young Green Coconut Milk

Up until a few years ago, the only time I saw a green coconut was on vacation, with a straw in it. Little did I know I would be hacking ... I mean, cracking them open every week like I work on a beach! I use young green coconuts mainly for the water they contain. This younger variety has more nutrients, electrolytes, protein, B vitamins, minerals, and other goodies our hair, mind, and body love.

If you drink or cook with its contents, the healing goodness that comes from this bodacious botanical is powerful enough to:

1. Cleanse your liver (rules the skin, joints, and eyes)
2. Prevent and heal digestive disorders
3. Help you lose weight
4. Clear and naturally enhance your complexion—helps skin tags, moles, and brown spots fade away[36]

I specifically use coconut water to make a dairy-free probiotic drink that helps my seven-year-old improve his speech and communication, and strengthens his immune system. As a result, I have young green coconuts all over the place and lots of coconut meat left over.

Of course you don't have to crack open a coconut to make this recipe; I have two coconut milk recipes for you. One is more intense than the other, but both make a delicious coconut milk. You can also buy some pretty healthy, store bought versions if making them is not your thing… but give it a try!

For how to make your own coconut milk from young green coconuts watch my *How To Make Coconut Milk Video* on YouTube.com/EricaKTV. You can also access this video at EricaKKing.com/coconutmilk.

Coconut Milk Quickie | **Raw Chocolate Milk Shake**

Ingredients

1 1/2 cup coconut milk
1 teaspoon cocoa powder
1/2 teaspoon matcha green tea
1/4 teaspoon maca root powder
1/4 teaspoon raw agave syrup
1/2 cup ice
A really cool straw

Instructions

1. Add coconut milk, matcha green tea, cocoa powder, raw agave syrup and ice to a high speed blender.
2. Blend on high for up to 1 minute.
3. Get a really cool straw and enjoy!

Sesame Seed Milk

This alkaline food will help keep your body's pH levels in check. Sesame seeds are also incredibly rich in calcium, which supports bone growth, helps ease migraines, and can relieve symptoms of PMS. Drinking sesame seed milk will also provide you with a healthy dose of magnesium, copper, vitamin B1, zinc, and dietary fiber. This milk is extremely healthy and contains loads of calcium.

Ingredients

1 cup sesame seeds
2 1/2 cups water
4 pitted dates
1/2 teaspoon vanilla extract
fine mesh strainer or nut milk bag
32 ounce jar or pitcher with lid

Instructions

1. Turn your oven to 400 degrees. Roast the sesame seeds for 10 minutes. Remove from the oven and allow to cool for a few minutes.
2. Add water and sesame seeds to your blender and blend on the highest speed for up to 5 minutes.
3. Pour your sesame seed milk through the strainer until no pulp remains. You may have to repeat this process a few times.
4. Once the pulp has been removed, pour the sesame seed milk back into the blender. Add dates and vanilla extract. Blend on high for up to 2 minutes, or until your milk is smooth.
5. Pour the milk through the strainer again to remove any remaining pulp. Store your milk in a 32 ounce container with lid.

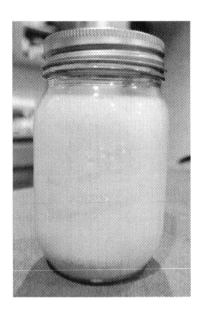

Sunflower Seed Milk

Sunflower seed milk is a delicious, creamy option to add to your milk substitutes. It has a milk, slightly nutty taste that reminds you a little of almond milk. High in vitamin E, which is wonderful for our hair and skin, this milk is also high in the mineral selenium, which is great for a healthy metabolism. Here's a quick recipe:

Erica's Sunflower Seed Milk Recipe

3 cups water
1 cup raw sunflower seeds
1 teaspoon vanilla
1 tablespoon maple syrup
For a sugar-free option: substitute 3 drops vanilla cream stevia for maple syrup

Instructions

1. Blend on high for up to 1 minute or until the milk is smooth.
2. Strain any remaining sunflower seeds from the milk before adding vanilla and sweetner.

Sweet Flax Milk

Flax milk contains omega-3 fatty acids from cold-pressed flax oil that has been shown to help prevent diabetes, heart disease cancer, and strokes. It contains no saturated or trans fat and is fortified with minerals and vitamins, including vitamins A, B12, and D, as well as calcium. Creamy, tasty, versatile and packed full of nutrients and fiber, it is one of the newer milk alternatives to be commercially available that is rapidly gaining popularity.

If you like discovering natural products, you've probably heard someone mention flaxseeds at some point. There are flaxseed gels, conditioners, even my personal favorite, the crunchy salad topping, but have you ever had flaxseed milk?

I know, not your typical first choice for milk. But in my home, nut milks are out (two nut allergies), cow's milk is no good (one food sensitivity), and it needs to taste good sugar-free for my son's treatment and recovery.

Coconut milk and hempseed milk are our favorites, and when I saw flax milk in my local farmer's market, I couldn't wait to try making my own. It's the perfect milk substitute whenever you want more vitamins, fiber, and nutrients added to your meals.

Flaxseeds are about two dollars per pound, easy to find, and can be used as an egg replacer, deep conditioner, and hair growth booster! As awesome as these seeds are for your hair, it's what they do for your body that's even more spectacular!

Flaxseeds reduce the risk of:

- heart disease
- cancer
- stroke
- diabetes

What makes flaxseeds so good for you?

It's their omega-3 essential fatty acids, lignans, and fiber! Each tablespoon has 1.8 grams of omega-3. Lignans are phytonutrients that help regulate hormones.

They contain plant estrogen and antioxidants that help with:

- hair growth
- breast health
- diabetes
- ovarian and uterine health
- relief from menopause

Recipe Essentials:

flaxseeds (brown)
nut milk bag or strainer
purified water
sealable jar, container, or pitcher for milk

Sweet Flax Milk Ingredients

1/3 cup flaxseeds
4 cups of water
3 whole dates (pitted)
1 teaspoon vanilla

Instructions

1. Add water and flaxseeds to high-speed blender.
2. Blend the ingredients on high for up to a minute or until smooth.
3. Use the nut milk bag or strainer to remove any remaining flaxseeds.
4. After straining, add 3 whole dates (pitted).

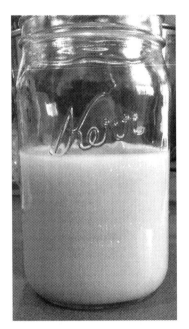

Sweet Flax Milk

Hemp Seed Milk

An 8-ounce glass of hemp seed milk contains all ten essential amino acids, 900 milligrams of omega-3 fatty acid, 4 grams of digestible protein, and copious amounts of riboflavin, phosphorous, vitamin A, and potassium. This gives us "softer skin, shinier hair, and stronger nails" (McKierman, 2021).

Hemp's anti-inflammatory agents help to strengthen the immune system and increase circulation. With its amazingly nutritious, light nutty flavor, it will fill you with essential amino acids, loads of vitamins and minerals, and a good dose of omega-3.

This is one of the few allergy-free milks that taste good fresh, without adding sweeteners. You may not want to chug a full glass, but you could. For a tasty recipe made with hemp seed milk, try the chia seed cereal at the end of this chapter!

Ingredients

1/2 cup organic raw, shelled hemp seeds
4 cups water

Instructions

Add the raw hemp seeds to your blender. Any blender will work. Blend on high-speed for 2 to 4 minutes. You may not have any actual seeds left in your milk. If you do have seeds left over, strain them from the milk. You can use a mesh strainer or nut bag (pour the milk through and squeeze the bag). If you're using a specialty blender (e.g., Blend-Tec, Vitamix), blend the milk on high for up to 1 minute.

Pour your milk in a pitcher or something with a lid. Hemp seed milk will last in the refrigerator for 3 to 5 days.

Where to Buy the Best Raw Hemp Seeds

I use the Manitoba Harvest Brand (Organic Hemp Hearts Raw Shelled Hemp Seeds). I buy them from Amazon because they last forever, stay fresh for a couple of months (in the refrigerator), and taste really good. There are lots of great organic options available at your local grocery. Check there and Amazon for more.

Guilt-Free Chia Seed Cereal with Maple Syrup

1/4 cup chia seeds
3 cups hemp seed milk
1 tablespoon cacao nibs
1 tablespoon lucuma powder
1/4 cup mulberries
1 teaspoon vanilla powder
1/2 teaspoon maple syrup
1/8 teaspoon vanilla creme stevia
1/2 teaspoon apple pie spice
1/2 teaspoon lemon juice
optional: diced fresh fruit

Instructions

1. Add chia seeds to your mixing bowl.
2. Slowly stir in 2 cups of milk. Keep stirring so the chia seeds do not clump together.
3. Add cacao nibs, lucuma powder, and mulberries and stir. Add in 1/4 cup more of the milk.
4. Stir in vanilla powder, maple syrup, stevia, apple spice, and lemon juice.
5. This cereal will thicken as it sits. Gradually add in remaining milk.
6. Sit the cereal in the refrigerator for 20 minutes.
7. Stir, top with fresh fruit (pineapples are great), and enjoy!

Chapter 13

The Beginner's Guide to Juicing

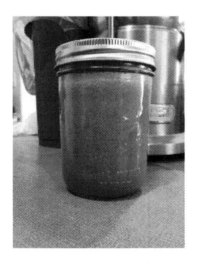

"Virtually all vegetables can be juiced, as well as fruits. You should aim to drink between three and four green vegetables per week. The best juicing vegetables include watercress, parsley, spinach, zucchini, green peppers and lettuce. As fruits are high in fructose, it is advisable to dilute fruit juices 50% with water."
Vicki Edgson and Ian Marber, The Food Doctor—
Healing Foods for Mind and Body

Have you ever made your own fruit juice? Have you ever watched those juicing infomercials where they stuff a whole apple into the juicer and almost a full glass of apple juice appears?

Juicing is one of the key elements in a holistically healthy lifestyle. Why? Juicing allows you to get all of the vitamins, minerals, and pure water from fruits and plants for instant nutrition. Nutritional therapists have used juicing and concentrated vitamin and mineral supplements in the treatment of cancer, high blood pressure, autoimmune diseases, autism, and other chronic conditions.

Freshly squeezed orange juice is no comparison to store bought. Blueberry juice is unbelievably good, and pear juice is the base for mostly all store-bought juices you consume.

Check the label!

Here are some important points to remember:

- Vegetable juices build and regenerate.
- Fruit juices cleanse.
- Use carrot and celery for the base of your vegetable juices (although carrots can also be used in fruit juice).
- Add an apple for flavor.
- Add lemon to water and any juice to cleanse.

For more energy:

Juice carrots, spinach, kale, cabbage, grapefruit, celery, peppers of all colors (green, red, orange, yellow), parsley, and ginger.

For less stress:

Juice carrots, spinach, celery, lettuce, broccoli, celery, beets, cilantro, and wheatgrass.

Add to any juice recipe:

Carrots are good for your liver, skin, intestines, and eyes and to cure ulcers. Celery is a nerve tonic. It helps cleanse the blood, improves taste, and boosts energy.

Cucumbers are packed with Vitamin A and E. It's a natural diuretic that's great for lowering blood pressure, and improving skin, hair, and nails.

Romaine lettuce is good brain food, helps improve concentration, and is also good for your eyes.

Parsley helps clear arteries, eliminates cramps, and is good for your eyes and kidneys.

Spinach helps with healthy gums, soothes and cleanses your entire intestinal tract, and fights anemia.

Wheatgrass protects and builds the muscles, glands, and tissues of the body.[52]

Recipe Extra | *All-Natural Fruit and Veggie Wash*

Don't forget to wash your veggies before drinking. This will remove any leftover pesticides, toxins, dirt, grime, and critters who may still be enjoying the goods.

3 cups water (or fill a sink with water)
2 tablespoons apple cider vinegar
2 tablespoons lemon juice
1 tablespoon baking soda

Instructions:

1. Add the vinegar, lemon juice, and soda to water. I like to use the sink. Soak as many fruits and vegetables that will fit. If you need to turn them or move them around, go ahead. I like to press my green leafies down a few times, as they will usually rise to the top of the water.
2. Once you add your produce, let them sit in the wash for at least 30 minutes.
3. Rinse your fruit and veggies individually and don't be afraid to use a veggie brush to get off any lingering dirt. You'll be surprised at what you find left in the sink.

Note

Even and especially if you buy organic, make sure to wash anything you eat or juice.

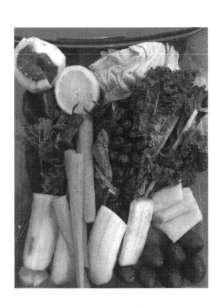

Best Raw Living Foods for Hair Growth

By Emily Cedar, Health and Wellness Activist, Naturalista

Incorporating raw living foods into your diet is one of the healthiest and most effective ways to repair damaged hair and stimulate its growth. Eating foods rich in antioxidants like vitamin C and E will take your beauty regimen to a whole new level. Let's dive into the food sources and benefits of these powerful vitamins and minerals.

Stimulate Hair Growth and Repair Damaged Follicles

Vitamin C is an all-star antioxidant because it aids in the formation of collagen while absorbing iron. This combination helps fight hair loss and leads to healthy, luscious locks. Unfortunately, the human body cannot produce vitamin C on its own, so it's vital to incorporate the foods that are packed with this good stuff into your daily diet. Great sources of vitamin C include oranges, papaya, tangerines, pineapple, broccoli, cucumbers, bell peppers, and dark leafy greens.

Vitamin E is another antioxidant that packs a lot of punch. It repairs damaged follicles, rebuilds tissue, and deeply conditions hair from the roots to the ends. These stellar features of vitamin E prevent premature graying and boost hair growth. To reap the benefits of this vitamin, incorporate foods like sunflower seeds, kiwi, hazelnuts, asparagus, spinach, almonds, avocado, and Swiss chard into your diet.

In addition to fueling yourself with vitamins E and C, supplement your diet with plenty of antioxidant compounds. These are known to prevent and slow cell damage while increasing blood flow and improving circulation to the body and scalp. Over time, this leads to more consistent and healthier hair growth. Antioxidant-rich foods are plentiful and can be easily packed into a colorful salad. Some of my favorites are strawberries, beets, blueberries, tomatoes, and eggplants.

Prevent and Release Breakage

Foods filled with healthy fats, omega-3 fatty acids, protein, calcium, iron, and B vitamins moisturize hair and prevent breakage and dryness. Some of the best foods for this are chia seeds, almonds, cacao, acai, avocados, and walnuts.

Chia seeds are a great source of calcium, iron, and B vitamins. *Cacao* is rich in iron, zinc, and magnesium, making it an excellent option for promoting long and strong hair. The *omega-3 fatty acids* in acai, avocados, and walnuts deeply hydrate and rejuvenate hair. Mix and match these foods to create a killer breakfast smoothie or chia seed pudding (see recipes below).

Recipes

Chia Seed Pudding: chia seeds, coconut milk, cacao, fresh mulberries, vanilla powder

Kale, Cucumber, and Beet Salad: olive oil, pink Himalayan salt, pepper, kale, beets, cucumbers

Green Smoothie: hemp seed milk, avocado, kale, spinach, banana, frozen blueberries, cinnamon

Tropical Fruit Salad: papaya, pineapple, tangerines, oranges, strawberries (sprinkle chia seeds on top as a bonus)

Drink the Rainbow | Juice Recipes for Naturals

Juicing is equally prevention and treatment in a glass. It provides healing and nourishment on all levels—spiritual, physical, mental, emotional, and psychological. We receive a bolus dose of vitamins and minerals that's difficult to achieve eating them one at a time.

The juice recipes in this section are all colors of the rainbow, and especially green juice! Green juice can help you relieve stress, strengthen your bones, improve mental clarity, and strengthen your intuition.

In my family, juicing has helped us reduce the effects or completely eliminate nasty cases of the flu, autism, severe eczema, dry, itchy skin, a weakened immune system, hair breakage, hair loss, and funky scalp (chlorine can be a beast). We've also raised test scores, dissolved sugar cravings, and developed a green thumb. You should try my wheatgrass!

What might these recipes hold for you? The healing is endless! I'm starting you off a juice legend. If you juice, she is bound to enter your kitchen and brighten your day. The green queen of juice, Green Goddess.

As a kale evangelist, it is my responsibility to tell you to go with dinosaur kale (lacinato kale, also referred to as Tuscan kale, cavolo nero) for this recipe. Its dark green, thick, coarse leaves are higher than other forms of kale in:

1. *Vitamin K (strong bones, teeth, and hair)*
2. *Vitamin A (great for cellular health, vision, and the reproductive system)*
3. *Vitamin C (big booster of the immune system)*

It's high in B vitamins (the feel-good vitamins), vitamin E (great for hair shine, volume, and growth), calcium (strengthens the heart), and fiber (keeps you feeling full and prosperous on all levels).

Green Goddess

What's in this juice?

Kale

I love kale because it's full of fiber, detoxifies your body, fights cancer, and adds a noticeable glow to your hair and skin. Kale is filled with nourishing nutrients, including vitamins K, A, C, B1, B2, B3, and B6.

Spinach

Spinach isn't lagging behind. She's filled with vitamins, K, A, B2, B3, and B6, omega-3 fats, iron, and more marvelous minerals. Helping ease digestion and elimination, she and her BFF kale are power foods that will help deepen your feelings of relaxation.

Cucumber

Cucumber also detoxifies. It's a natural diuretic, wonderful for your hair and skin, and has an extremely mild taste. A cucumber always adds way more juice than you think it can hold. Peel your cucumbers unless you buy organic. The skin is awesome (filled with bodacious nutrients and goodies), but nonorganic can be heavily sprayed with toxic pesticides.

Apples

Apples will sweeten any juice, so if you don't like a green full-bodied taste (or if green juice makes you gag), add an apple. Granny Smiths are best because they add sweetness and not too much sugar to your beverage. Use stevia to sweeten if needed. Start with one drop; it's three hundred times more potent than sugar.

Ginger

Ginger will stop an upset stomach on the spot and intensify your prosperity experience! If you love ginger, use as much as you're used to. It has a relaxing effect on your digestive system and is very soothing overall.

Lemons

Lemons are amazing. They liven up your drink, make it a little more refreshing, and allow you to keep the extras in your refrigerator overnight without it turning to gunk.

Green Goddess

Ingredients

3 big kale leaves and stems
1 fistful of spinach
1 cucumber
1 Granny Smith apple
1 lemon
1/4 ginger (about the size of a thumb:)

Instructions

1. Wash and prepare your fruit and veggies.
2. Run your ingredients through your juicer.
3. Pour, stick a straw in, and go.

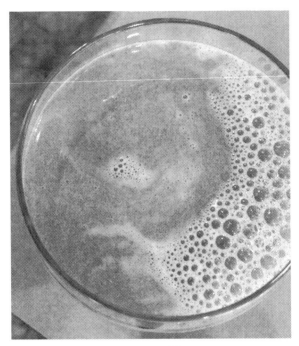

Green Goddess

Joyful Greens

Ingredients

4 kale leaves and stems
1 cucumber
3 apples
handful of spinach
handful of cilantro
1 celery stalk

Instructions

1. Wash and prep all ingredients.
2. Run them through your juicer in the order listed.

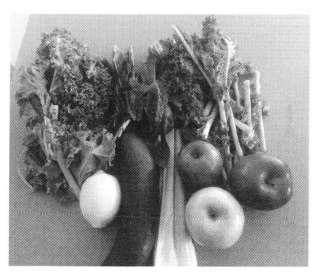

Joyful Greens

Pineapple Green

There are a few ingredients that are always my green basics.

Kale, cucumber, and spinach usually make up 95 percent of most green juices. The fancy folks may also include celery, Swiss chard, parsley, and cilantro. I usually juice what's in my refrigerator after my latest fruit and veggie haul.

Which is how I came up with this recipe. I ran out of spinach and parsley (I'm fancy) and didn't want the strong taste of celery, so I decided to juice what was left—green beans. Because I was unsure, I decided to go heavy on my fruit, which means a heavier concentration of sugar. If you're watching your sugar intake, you may want to dilute your juice with fresh water before drinking.

Watch the throwback video for this recipe on EricaKTV: http://youtu.be/zkUeGumTf6E.

Ingredients

1/2 pineapple
1 orange
1 carrot
1/2 cucumber
handful of kale
handful of green beans

Instructions

1. Wash and prep all ingredients.
2. Run them through your juicer in the order listed.

Heart Chakra

Ingredients

1 orange
1 pear
2 cucumbers
1 carrot
handful of spinach
2 kale leaves with stems
1/2 lemon

Instructions

1. Wash and prep all ingredients.
2. Run ingredients through your juicer.
3. Pour and enjoy!

Authentic Self

Wisdom, higher states of consciousness, and peace are a few effects of Authentic Self. Served over ice, you won't know whether you're drinking a fresh, juicy punch or the natural wine from heaven!

If there was an award for best green juice taste, this one would win! It tastes like a juicy punch with fruits and veggies that love being together. You can tell! There are lots of Green Goddess recipes. If you juice long enough (over a day), you'll make up one of your own!

Ingredients

1/2 pineapple
big ole' fistful of kale
big ole' fistful of spinach
1 cucumber
1 orange
1 mango
1 nectarine

Instructions

1. Cleanse and prep your ingredients.
2. Juice them while doing a happy dance.

Green Diva

Getting my kids (two, four, and six at the time) to drink a green juice in the beginning … pure comedy.

Until the ultimate smoothie.

This pineapple-strawberry smoothie is so good you won't believe it's green. There's no better way to get the mega vitamins A, C, K, potassium, and calcium (to name a few) in your system. After a few minutes, you can literally feel it in your bones!

Green Diva is more of a juice with luscious pulp. It's very frothy and slightly thick. Even with ice cubes it can have a smoothie type of texture. This juice is naturally sweet. There's no need for stevia or honey. The succulence of your mango and sweet tartness of the pineapple will make you feel like you're enjoying this one on the beach!

Green Diva Recipe

Ingredients

1 mango
1 orange
6 strawberries
1/4 pineapple
handful of kale with stems
handful of spinach with stems
1 cucumber

Instructions

1. Wash, prep, and peel your ingredients.
2. Run them through your juicer with a smile.
3. Serve over ice.

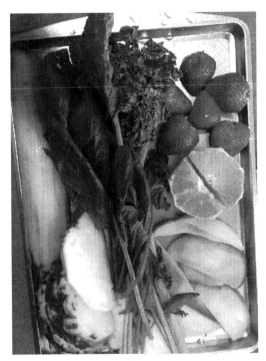

Green Diva Ingredients

Swiss Papaya

Ingredients

1/2 lemon
1/2 papaya
1/4 cabbage
2 Swiss chard leaves with stems
1 cucumber
Optional: 1 apple for sweetness

Instructions

1. Wash and peel your ingredients.
2. Run them through your juicer.

This juice is a veggie lover's dream!

It's packed full of vitamins C and K, electrolytes, calcium, potassium, riboflavin, and a bunch of other essentials you're used to seeing on the bottle of a multivitamin ... and that's just from the cabbage!

It contains amino acids like glutamine (Swiss chard and stems), which helps the body heal and boosts the immune system. Other benefits of this beverage are:

- *contains lots of fiber*
- *good for your brain*
- *high in sulfur*
- *great for your waist line*

It is not, however, great on taste if you like sweeter-tasting juices. Even with the delicious papaya and orange, it has a stronger veggie-ish taste than most drinks. I love the taste of this version, but you can always add more citrus, a whole papaya instead of half, an apple, or stevia drops to sweeten.

The Sugar Crusher

The purpose of this drink is to stop sugar in its tracks. My red velvet cake lovers, my krispy kreme peeps, and all of you hard candy buffs, late-night sugar cravings can expand your midsection, keep you up at night, and cause feelings of sadness, mental fogginess, and in some cases depression.

The Sugar Crusher is high in calcium, magnesium, manganese, phosphorus, potassium, trace minerals zinc and selenium. Each of these is important for a healthy, heart and healthy immune system.

Wheatgrass is a wonderful, revitalizing source of balanced nutrients for the mind and body. It's a source of all B vitamins, including folic acid, pantothenic acid, choline, and a vegetable source of B-12.[52]

Ingredients

fistful of wheatgrass
handful of cilantro
handful of parsley
2 carrots
1 apple
1/4 beet
1/2 lemon

Instructions

1. Wash and prep your goodies.
2. Run them through your juicer in the order listed.
3. Drink while reciting the following prayer: "Create in me a pure heart holy spirit; renew a right spirit within me."

Hallelujah Morning Detox

Ingredients

1/2 pineapple
1/2 lemon
3 kale leaves with stems
a big handful of cilantro
1 cucumber

Instructions

1. Run your ingredients through your juicer.
2. Drink Hallelujah within 15 minutes for maximum benefits.
3. This juice can be stored up to 12 hours in the refrigerator.

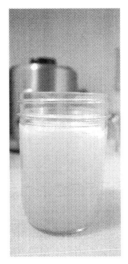

Perfect Papaya Pineapple

Perfect Papaya Pineapple

An any-day favorite during all seasons! The perfect juice for breakfast, lunch, or dinner. It's so naturally sweet you won't taste the cabbage, cucumber, or spinach that give this juice the greens you need!

Ingredients

1/2 papaya
1 pear
1/4 of a whole pineapple (or 1 cup)
1/4 cabbage
1 cucumber
3 handfuls of spinach

Instructions

1. Wash, peel, and prep your ingredients,
2. Run them through your juicer and enjoy!

Papaya and her seeds contain papain. This enzyme helps reduce inflammation. One study showed consuming papain reduces indigestion. Referred to as "fruit of the angels," the B vitamins in papayas help balance mood and improve concentration and the quality of your sleep.

Papaya is filled with:

- vitamin A
- vitamin C *(224% of the recommended daily intake)*
- folate
- calcium
- potassium
- iron
- thiamin
- fiber
- magnesium
- pantothenic acid

Juice Tip:

If you're using home-grown veggies, leave the skin on for more nutrients, vitamins, and minerals.

Body Glow

When we moved to Maui for my husband's job a few years ago, I had my choice of exotic fruits and vegetables right outside my front door. It was as close to juicing in heaven as I've ever been! Fresh organic papayas were so plentiful there they were often given away (they ripen super fast) or less than a quarter!

I created this recipe after a day at the Baby Beach (Maui's Baldwin Beach Park) without sunscreen. Let's just say, body glow is a healing beverage that speeds the healing of skin and tastes great at the beach! It's a full-bodied green drink with lots of sweetness. Packed with body- and skin-loving ingredients that give you energy and a beautiful glow!

Ingredients

1 papaya
1 cucumber
1 pear
1/4 cabbage
3 handfuls of spinach

Instructions

1. Wash, peel, and prep your ingredients.
2. Juice and enjoy!

If you're using organic, you may leave the skin on. The skin of the papaya is super rich in vitamins, minerals, and nutrients.

Here are some additional benefits of Body Glow's delicious ingredients:

Spinach

Packed with vitamins A, K, C, and the feel-good B vitamins (B1, B2, B3, and B6), the three handfuls of spinach in this blend will awaken your body and keep your energy balanced all day (no midday crash)! It's also a great source of iron and fiber.

Vitamin A helps with cell growth, boosting your immune system, and keeping your skin healthy and vibrant. It also promotes healthy teeth, soft tissue, protects your mucus membranes, and promotes healthy vision. This pro-vitamin also helps maintain the health of your reproductive organs.

Vitamin K is actually a group of fat-soluble compounds (K, K1, K2, K3) that help the body recover from injuries and prevent excessive bleeding. These vitamin compounds also help carry calcium throughout the body. This helps prevent bone loss and fractures. Vitamin K is most known for its ability to help blood clot normally, making this one of the first vitamin shots given to newborns.

Papaya

Sweet papayas are full of vitamins A and C, as well as lots of minerals, antioxidants, enzymes, and nutrients. The vitamins and minerals in papaya help prevent heart disease, slow the development and growth of cancer, and weaken the effects of aging. My favorite benefit: they help balance blood sugar and provide enough energy for you for the day!

Pear

This funky fresh fruit is high in fiber and vitamins C and E. Some of its other delicious health benefits include:

- reduces high blood pressure
- lowers cholesterol

- has more pectin than an apple, which means it's excellent to relieve constipation (pectin acts as a mild laxative and diuretic)
- a great source of energy
- supports bone health, reducing the risk of osteoporosis
- boosts the immune system
- reduces the risk of type 2 diabetes
- helps reduce cancer risk

Cucumber

Packed with the beloved feel-good B vitamins, I find it hard to juice without adding at least a half a cucumber to my blends. Cucumbers are excellent to add to any fruit juice. They have hardly any taste and hold more water than you'd think.

Its powerful anti-inflammatory properties make this a very gentle, natural diuretic that keeps your belly and intestines happy!

Cucumbers contain:

- vitamin C
- beta-carotene
- manganese
- flavonoids, lignans, and triterpenes (a group of compounds and phytonutrients that have been found to fight and reduce the risk of breast cancer and cancer of the uterus, ovaries, and prostate)

Pineapple Orange Juice

Ingredients

1 to 2 oranges
1/2 pineapple
1/2 lime
2 carrots
1/4 cabbage
1 kale leaf
1 1/4 cucumbers

Instructions

1. Cleanse and prep your ingredients.
2. Run them through the juicer in the order presented.
3. Pour them in your glass or cup and enjoy!

Optional

Leave out the cabbage and add 1/4 sweet potato and 1/2 mango!

Cabbage reduces belly fat, it's full of fiber, and it calms the digestive system. It naturally detoxifies the body and lifts a low mood.

Sweet Pineapple Juice

Add a little sweetness to your day with Sweet Pineapple Juice. It's packed with veggies and taste. This recipe includes another super food that will add extra fiber (keeps you full) and nutrients to your system.

Sweet potatoes are abundantly filled with vitamins A, C, and B6, fiber, calcium, and magnesium (a natural muscle relaxer). This super food helps keep your blood pressure in check, boosts your iron levels, strengthens your bones, and speeds up your metabolism. Pretty sweet!

Ingredients

1/2 pineapple
1 orange
1/2 cucumber
4 kale leaves
1/2 sweet potato

Instructions

1. Cleanse and prep your ingredients.
2. Juice or blend with a smile.

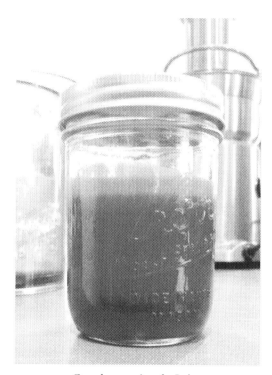

Cranberry Apple Juice

Cranberry Apple Juice

http://lavishlynatural.com/cranapplejuice/

Ingredients

1 cup cranberries
2 apples
1/2 lemon
3 carrots
1/4 beet
small handful of collard greens
1 cucumber

Instructions

1. Wash and prep all ingredients.
2. Run fruit and vegetables through juicer.

This juice is both sweet and tart but mostly sweet! If you experience a midday energy zap and reach for coffee, juice this instead.

Cranberry Apple Juice benefits:

- relieves stress
- boosts immune system
- shrinks and eliminates the growth of tumors
- removes heavy metals from the blood
- good for skin
- calms the digestive system
- prevents blood clots
- strengthens bones
- tastes too good to have a beet in it

Green juices are popular, but it's the rainbow of colors that keeps you healthy and awesome! If you've heard of the Green Goddess, (or if you enjoy my pretty Green Goddess), get your taste buds ready!

Red Goddess is a blend of beetroot, beet greens, spinach, and cucumber. Don't run for the door yet. This juice is naturally sweetened by the beets themselves and fresh carrots, pear, and a little lemon and lime.

Beet greens can be a little bitter, so the lemon and lime do an excellent job of eliminating any bitter taste. The pear adds a heap of sweetness! You may also add your sweetener of choice (1 to 2 teaspoons) if you want a little more.

It's worth it to have these greens in your system—raw! Beet greens contain more nutrients than the beetroot itself. They also have more iron in them than spinach. Substitute beet greens for lettuce on your sandwiches. Add a little to your salads and of course, to your green drinks!

Beets are:

- filled with fiber
- a great source of protein, zinc, and phosphorus
- rich in antioxidants
- helpful for improving blood pressure
- high in magnesium, potassium, copper, and manganese
- packed with vitamin B6 (the feel-good vitamin that improves mood), vitamin K, and vitamin C
- a good source of iron and calcium
- known to have an anti-inflammatory effect on the body

Beet greens contain a bodacious dose of vitamin A (220 percent of the daily recommended intake), which boosts the immune system, encourages eye health, and improves our reproductive system.

Vitamin A:

- reduces heavy menstrual flow
- helps relieve yeast infections
- relieves the symptoms of PMS
- speeds healing from vaginal infections
- raises sperm count

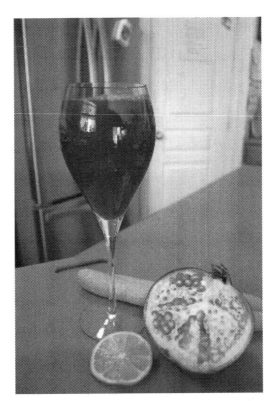

Pomegranate Punch

Pomegranate Punch

Ingredients

1 apple
1 pomegranate
1/2 lime
1 carrot
small handful of cilantro
1/2 cucumber
1 kale leaf with stem
1 turnip green leaf with stem

Instructions

1. Wash and prep all ingredients.
2. Run ingredients through juicer.

Pomegranate juice helps improve blood flow to the heart, which reduces the risks associated with heart disease.

Pomegranate juice also:

- helps stop plaque buildup in blood vessels
- decreases LDL cholesterol
- slows the growth of prostate cancer
- contains high amounts of three different types of antioxidants: polyphenols, anthocyanins, and ellagic acid (these micronutrients help your body resist cellular damage, aging, and inflammation)

Bluepeary Apple Juice

Ingredients

1/4 cup blueberries (fresh)
1 apple
1 pear
1 cucumber
3 kale leaves with stems

Instructions

1. Wash, prep, and peel your ingredients.
2. Run ingredients through your juicer.
3. Drink within 15 minutes for maximum nutrient and vitamin absorption … although anytime is a good time for green juice!

Ingredient Spotlight: Blueberries

Blueberries are packed with many nutrients and minerals, including the following:

- vitamin C boosts your immune system
- vitamin E: helps prevent cancer; essential for healthy skin
- vitamin A: good for healthy skin, eyes, bones, and immune function
- niacin: helps convert food into energy
- riboflavin: helps keep your skin and eyes healthy
- potassium: a mineral that's good for regulating blood pressure, water balance, muscles, nerves, and digestion
- manganese: essential trace mineral that helps metabolize fat and proteins
- fiber: good for a healthy digestive system

Green Buddha

This recipe comes from my son, Damon. He's not a huge fan of green juice, even though he drinks it almost every day. So when I find out that he wants more (like he's drinking a juicy juice), I take notice and quickly write down the ingredients!

This is one of those recipes ... and it's made with our favorite sugar-free, non-blood-sugar-raising stevia!

Woohoo!

What is stevia?

Stevia is a plant-based sweetener and sugar substitute that is about three hundred times sweeter than sugar. A little will go around the world and back, so start with one drop and gradually increase. When buying this luscious sweetener, read the product label carefully. It should be 100 percent pure, with no added ingredients.

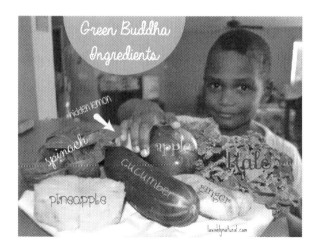

Green Buddha Recipe

Light, sweet, and refreshing. Balance your mood, increase weight loss, improve the quality of your sleep, and experience a deeper level of mental clarity—one sip at a time.

Ingredients

1/4 ginger
1/4 pineapple
1/4 lemon
1 apple
a big handful of spinach

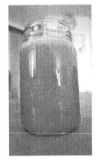

Green Buddha

Instructions

1. Wash, prep, and peel ingredients in the order listed (sweetest ingredients first).
2. Run the ingredients through your juicer.
3. Drink and repeat this hair affirmation: my word creates my world.

Juice Tip:

This juice is sweet enough with the pineapple, but I like ginger and apple together. If you are seeking more sugar-free options to sweeten your juice, consider adding low-glycemic fruit stevia. I use sweet leaf stevia (lemon drop). Download this recipe and benefits at http://ericakking. com/greenbuddha/.

Abundance

This green juice is its own prosperity practice!

It's got kale, cucumber, spinach (my juice trifecta), pear, ginger, lemon, and cabbage. An abundance of greens and nutrients that literally help you release old ideas, thoughts, feelings, memories, patterns, and conditions from your body.

Benefits from this bountifully green beverage:

- *promotes mental clarity and emotional balance*
- *increases awareness*
- *improves the ability to concentrate*
- *dissolves fear*
- *boosts energy and confidence*
- *helps release stress and feelings of overwhelm from your joints, muscles, and bones*
- *increases feelings of relaxation*
- *creates good energy and balance in the brain, body*

Taste Review

This juice is surprisingly sweet. There's just enough ginger for a teeny-weeny bit of spice but not so much that it overpowers the juice. For as many greens that are in this, you really can't tell by the taste.

A deeply "green" juice packed with abundance, prosperity, and total fulfillment. Drinking this will attract more love, more wealth, and more health to your mind and body!

Ingredients

1/4 cabbage
3 kale leaves and stem
1 big handful of spinach
1/4 inch of ginger
1/4 lemon
1 pear

Instructions

1. Wash, prep, and peel your ingredients.
2. Juice or blend and sip!

Summer Peach Slushie

Ingredients

1/2 cup water
2 ripe peaches (peeled and pitted)
1/4 chopped mango (peeled and chopped)
1 tablespoon raw agave syrup
1 cup ice cubes

Instructions

1. Add water, peaches, mango, raw agave syrup and ice cubes to your high speed blender.
2. Blend on highest speed for up to 1 minute.

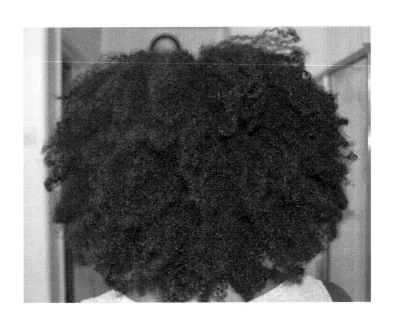

Chapter 14

Green Juice Recipes for Mental Wellness

"Every great drink starts with a plant."
Amy Stewart, The Drunken Botanist: The Plants
That Create The World's Great Drinks

Our busy schedules, constant states of information overload, and overstimulated brains leave most of us living with a mental fog surrounding us at all times. This fog limits our creativity and decision-making abilities, diverts our focus, and weighs us down both mentally and emotionally. Fortunately, there exists a natural solution to lifting mental fog that doesn't involve pills, surgery, or a fat wallet.

There are tons of mental and emotional benefits to juicing and drinking fresh fruits and vegetables.

According to the US National Library of Medicine, people who consume natural juice more than three times per week are 76 percent less likely to develop Alzheimer's disease than those who consume juice less than once a week. Not only will consuming natural juice help you maintain a healthy brain, but it will also allow you to become a more mindful, focused, and overall happier person.

Here's how...

Purify Your Mental and Emotional State
by Emily Cedar, Health and Wellness Activist, Naturalista
Juice Recipes by Ileana Piñero, Holistic Therapist, Chef, and Reiki Goddess

Drinking a glass of juice in the morning allows your body to absorb the nutrients it needs to heal itself, without bombarding it with toxins and hard-to-digest foods. Giving your digestive system a little break allows your body to focus on the areas that need healing. It helps strengthen our memory, boosts mental concentration, and lifts the mental fog that can cloud our judgment. The mind is typically one of first areas that needs a deep cleanse.

By consuming fresh juice, you not only eliminate harmful toxins from your body, but you also replace those impurities with brain-boosting nutrients. Apples are the perfect tasty ingredient for a morning juice and contain a powerful antioxidant called quercetin. Quercetin protects brain cells and prevents cognitive decline by shielding the brain from free radicals.

Similarly, by juicing leafy greens, you replenish the body with a healthy dose of vitamin K. Not only does vitamin K play a crucial role in fighting oxidative stress and maintaining the integrity of brain cells, but it has also been found to activate proteins crucial for brain function.

Try this green juice recipe for a purification and rejuvenation. It's wonderful for strengthing mental clarity and emotional balance.

Cucumber Passion

Benefits

This juice is rich in vitamin B6, folic acid, omega-3, antioxidants, and fiber. Cucumber juice is perfect to burn calories and lose weight so fast; for this you have to take it in the morning for ten consecutive days.

Ingredients:

1/2 lemon
2 pear
2 cucumber
1/2 celery
a small handful of fresh parsley (or 4 stems with leaves)
a small handful of fresh cilantro

Instructions

1. Wash, prep, and peel your ingredients.
2. Place your glass in the freezer for 15 minutes.
3. Run your ingredients through your juicer.
4. Pour your juice in your chilled glass and enjoy.

Expand Awareness and Cultivate Gratitude

By purifying the body and the brain, we are able create more space for mindfulness and gratitude. By simply noticing the foods that we put into our body, we bring a new level of awareness into our daily life; we become more mindful of how we do what we do. We are much more inclined to listen to our bodies and respond to what they need, instead of what the advertisements on television tell us to crave.

Listening to the true needs of our body is in itself an act of self-love.

By practicing self-love, we open the doors to a whole new realm of gratitude. Not only will you start to cultivate gratitude for the nourishment your juice gives your mind and body, but you will more easily express gratitude toward the simple things in life. Often times, these small, simple things are the most beautiful and yet the most overlooked.

Love Magnet

Benefits

- provides the body with phytonutrients, as well as a wide variety of trace minerals (chard)
- boosts the immune system, reduces feelings of depression and anixiety (basil)
- prevents dehydration and promotes detoxification of the body (cucumber)
- healthy source of sugar (apple)

Ingredients

2 swiss chard leaves with stems
2 big basil leaves with stems (or a small handful)
1 cucumber

1 green apple
1/4 lemon

Instructions

1. Wash, prep, and peel your ingredients.
2. Place your glass in the freezer for 15 minutes.
3. Run your ingredients through your juicer.
4. Pour your juice in your chilled glass and enjoy.

Let Go of Negative Thoughts and Emotions

The physical benefits of cleansing and purifying the body with fresh fruit and vegetable juice are undeniably satisfying. As we restore the physical body, we begin to repair and restore the emotional body.

By clarifying our mental and physical states through juicing, we are granted access to deeply stored emotions that have been tucked away for weeks, months, and even years. When we uncover these emotions, it can sometimes feel uncomfortable or even somewhat painful. This is because we've hidden and ignored these grudges, resentments, and negative thoughts instead of confronting and releasing them. Letting go of these thoughts and emotions that no longer serve us is a key component to achieving spiritual growth and overall happiness.

Juice Recipe | Hint of Mint

Benefits:

- improves digestion and reduces internal inflammation (mint)
- detoxifies and purifies the blood (kale)
- hydrates and quenches thirst (celery and cucumber)

Ingredients

1 handful fresh mint
2 lacinato kale leaves and stems
1/2 stalk celery
1 green apple
a handful of grapes
1/4 lemon

Instructions

1. Wash, prep, and peel your ingredients.
2. Run them through your juicer with a smile.
3. Serve over ice.

Recipe Extra *(from Erica)*

Calm and Cool Sweet Orange Blend (for Healing Anger)

Ingredients

5 drops sweet orange oil
5 drops rose oil
5 drops lavender oil
1/4 cup sunflower oil

Instructions

1. Add the oils to a 2-ounce bottle. Gently shake the bottle to blend. Add a few drops to your bath.
2. You may also add 4 to 8 drops of this blend to 4 ounces of distilled water for a calm and cool spritz.

Increase Creativity and Intuition

Spark more ideas and allow your creativity to flow through you by indulging in a morning juice in place of a sugary latte. Green juices are one of the most effective ways to get the gears in your brain turning. Instead of the quick jolt of energy and ensuing crash that you get from a cup of coffee, green juice provides your body with sustained energy from vitamins and antioxidants. Other ingredients that help fuel brainpower include beets, kale, sprouts, and ginger.

A large part of our creativity comes from listening to our intuition, or inner voice of wisdom. When we listen to our bodies and feed them the nutrients they need, we begin to listen to our true self. It's hard to hear your own inner wisdom when you are bogged down by negative thoughts, mental fog, and stress.

Adding ingredients like spinach to your juice can help decrease stress. The high magnesium content in spinach helps regulate cortisol levels and bring about feelings of well-being. Before beginning a major project or having a big brainstorming session, add some of these stress-reducing fruits and veggies to your juice: oranges, berries, asparagus, and banana.

Tantric Kale

Benefits:

- hydrates your body and is a healthy source of carbohydrates and electrolytes
- detoxifies and purifies your blood
- heals and repairs the scalp
- calms the mind and digestive system
- gives your body a lot of phytonutrients, which help the immune system against disease (kale and spinach)
- boosts intuition
- healthy source of sugar

Tantric Kale Ingredients

1 big fistful of spinach
2 kale leaves and stems
1 apple
1/2 peeled lemon

Instructions

1. Wash, prep, and peel your ingredients.
2. Run them through your juicer.
3. Drink and visualize everything going your way.

Enhance Decision-Making Abilities

To make a quick and clear decision, we have to be able to approach an issue objectively. This means leaving our emotional attachments behind us. As stated above, juicing helps us become more in tune with our emotions, so when it comes time to make a decision, we can objectively face any problem.

Simply by being more aware and living closer to the present moment, we can approach the task at hand with more mental clarity and focus. In addition, since juicing encourages us to listen to our bodies more intently, we also strengthen our ability to listen to our gut instinct, or intuition.

Tapping into one's intuition, cultivating awareness, and facing a decision from an objective standpoint are all key components that help us make faster and overall better decisions. However, science has more to say on the subject of contemplating a decision. Researchers from Virginia Tech, Skidmore College, and the University of New Hampshire found that happier people make faster and more consistent decisions.

Although it's not a known fact that juicing will indefinitely make you happier, it's hard to ignore the positive effects listed above. As we've discussed, juicing plays a crucial role in reducing stress and cultivating gratitude. It would only make sense that when the mind and body are less stressed and more relaxed, anything is possible!

Kiwi Apple Mango

Benefits:

Loaded with hair-loving vitamins A and C, antioxidants, and nutrients that protect hair and skin from dryness.

This fruit-based juice:

- reduces inflammation
- helps prevent hair loss
- thickens hair
- improves scalp circulation
- helps keep skin vibrant and healthy
- stimulates hair growth
- revitalizes and tones skin

Ingredients:

1 orange
1 mango
1 apple
1 kiwi
2 carrots
1 cucumber

Optional: add 1 teaspoon of matcha green tea for an energy boost; or add 1 probiotic supplement for a probiotic boost

Instructions

1. Wash, prep, and peel your ingredients.
2. Run them through your juicer with a smile.

Chapter 15

How to Use Energy Medicine to Grow Your Hair: The Seven Primary Chakras

You are responsible first and foremost for your own healing. Check to see if you can experience the compassion you are trying to give away. As a healer you move into a healthier existence when truth becomes the lesson and the path, not the obstacle or the struggle (from "The Healer," p. 61).
—Zenju Earthlyn Manuel, Black Angel Cards

Most people have heard the word chakra, but what exactly does it mean? A vital and often ignored aspect of well-being comes from these mystical aspects of your body. Understanding how to balance and energize your chakras will boost well-being in a multitude of ways, and it is much easier than you think!

Chak-what?

The word chakra is a Sanskrit word that translates as "wheel," "disk," or "vortex." Chakras are vortices or interconnected energy centers found throughout the body acting as both receivers and transmitters of energy.

There are seven major chakras and 122 minor chakras within the physical body.[52] There are other chakras that are located outside of the body. All of the organs and tissues in our body are influenced by the chakra closest to them.

"The energy transmitted by the Chakras impact the physical, mental, emotional, and spiritual energy within the body. Specific thought patterns and emotional responses affect specific Chakras," and each chakra is influenced and affected by the others (INVISD, 2001). The energy of each chakra begins at the base of the spine and moves up toward the crown at the top of the head.

Though mainly invisible to the naked human eye, at least through the narrow frequency of light that most people can detect, chakras look like spinning vortices of energy, a little bit like the spinning galaxies and stars photographed by the Hubble telescope.

Esoteric Energies

Spiritual teachers, mystics, martial artists, energy workers, and some scientists agree there is a subtle energy that permeates our being and is intrinsic to our existence. This energy has been given many different names by many different traditions from around the world. The Indian Vedic texts refer to it as *prana*. In Japan and China, it is called qi and chi respectively. Vril is the word the Vikings used, and more modern labels are Orgone, coined by the Austrian psychoanalyst and scientist Wilhelm Reich, and The Force (yep, that's right, from *Star Wars*).

This energy, also referred to as life force energy, is essentially consciousness in its rawest form. It is bioelectric energy, meaning it is produced by the biological tissue within the body. One of the major functions chakras fulfill is to transmute this very powerful spiritual energy into energy that our bodies' systems can use safely. The chakras influence the organs, muscles, veins, and all the biological systems in your body.

In the same way that electricity from the main grid goes through a transformer to reduce its voltage to be safely used by appliances in your home, the chakras take pure, etheric life force energy (which is a bit like electricity) and translate it into energy that your body can use.

Physical Function

Each chakra has a unique role and can be said to represent a different level of spiritual reality. For example, the root chakra is associated with our most basic and primal needs, such as survival and procreation, whereas the crown chakra is associated with spiritual realization and the divine/ heavenly realms.

As we move up the chakra system, the life force energy is refined, from the denser, slower vibrating energy of the root chakra, becoming increasingly lighter and vibrationally higher as it is refined even more moving up the chakras.

This does not mean that any one of the chakras is more important than the others; they are all of equal importance and all need to be respected and looked after in order for you to function optimally. Having a strong root chakra without an opened crown chakra may result in a personality that is very egotistic or materialistically orientated and lacks a sense of spirituality or anything greater than itself.

Physically, the chakras all correspond to various glands and nerve centers within the body and sit on top of each other vertically in alignment with the spine. This is where the spiritual realities meet our physical one. If energy gets blocked in one of the chakras, this will affect our physical and mental health. For example, a urinary or kidney infection may be the result of a blockage in the sacral chakra. An energetic block in the throat chakra can manifest itself as a difficulty in socializing and communicating openly with others.

To become aware of your chakra, simply focus your attention on the area it occupies in your body. The more energy you put into thinking about your chakra, the stronger it becomes. This is a quirk of quantum physics; energy goes where attention flows!

The Seven Primary Chakras

Chakra	Sanskrit Name	Location	Color*	Associated Organs	Associated With
Root	Muladhara	The perineum (between the anus and genitals)	**Red**	Spine, kidneys, bladder	Base human needs, sexuality, grounding, stability
Sacral	Svadhisthana	Behind the genitals	**Orange**	Reproductive organs	Creativity, sexuality, relationships
Solar plexus	Manipura	Navel	**Yellow**	Pancreas, liver	Willpower
Heart	Anahata	The center of the chest	**Green**	Heart, lungs	Emotions
Throat	Vishuddha	The throat	**Blue**	Throat, thyroid gland	Communication
Third eye	Ajna	Between the eyebrows	**Indigo**	Pituitary gland, lower brain	Psychic awareness
Crown	Sahasrara	The crown of the head	**Violet/ White**	Pineal gland, upper brain	Spiritual connectivity

*Note: *The seven chakras are often depicted as corresponding to the seven colors of the rainbow; however, everyone's chakras are unique, and colors vary amongst individuals. Once you have started to work with your chakras, you might see them in your mind or even see hints of color around you, like an aura, especially in dim lighting.*

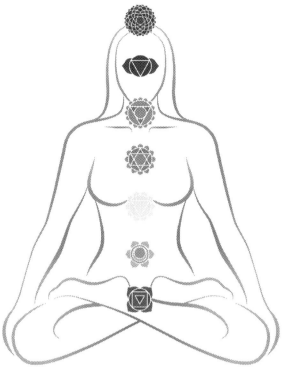

Crown Chakra

Third Eye Chakra

Throat Chakra

Heart Chakra

Solar Plexus Chakra

Sacral Chakra

Root Chakra

Going Within | The Chakra System and How to Use It

There is an unlimited number of healing methods. We'll test many of these ancient yet cutting-edge practices during the twenty-one-day diet. One of the most powerful systems of the body are the chakra.

Chakras may sound a bit funny, but they are glorious to work with. When you don't have the words to discuss what's happening, you can refer to your chakra to "diagnose" the situation.

You can use chakra colors to shift your mood. You can breathe into a seemingly unsolvable problem and get answers. You can literally watch it begin to change right before your eyes.

How?

Simply from knowing they exist and how they work. Keep in mind that the chakras manage the flow and energy centers of the body that influence the major organs, thoughts, ideas, emotions, beliefs, and behaviors. Our chakras even influence the foods we choose to eat.

The best way to understand the chakras is to use them. The chakra chart that follows presents the individual characteristics of each chakra and what heals it. You'll have a chance to work with a few of the chakras during the diet as well. One easy way is to surround yourself in the color of the chakra that you'd like to work with. Color therapy has been an effective method of healing for almost a century. It influences our physiological body (organs, tissues, blood flow, circulation), psychological health, and behavioral action. It's why you chose to wear that color you're wearing today. Marketers and advertisers use this research to get your attention and sell awesome products.

We're using them for healing, just like our ancestors.

How to Read the Chart

The chart highlights the following individual characteristics about each chakra:

- chakra name
- chakra color
- life experience and spiritual principle
- area of the body it manages
- treatments (healing breath, sound, and note)
- healing fruit, veggies, and juice
- healing oils, stones, and crystals

To heal, clear, or balance a chakra, read through the chart and see which chakra speaks to you. One, if not more, will usually jump out like "Pick me!"

If that doesn't happen, start with the root! I've included healing juice recipes for each chakra. Did you know that each chakra has its own healing oil and butter? Using shea butter in your hair products not only heals and moisturizes the skin, it also keeps your crown chakra in check—balanced and beautiful. Use the scent of rosemary, amber, or bergamot when working with the crown chakra. These scents make you more aware, cheerful, and at peace in your mind and body.

The Chakra Chart

Chakra	Life Experience and Spiritual Principle	Area of the Body	Treatments (Healing Breath, Sound, and Note)	Healing Fruit, Veggies, and Juice	Healing Oils, Stones, and Crystals
Crown Colors: violet, white, and gold	Awareness Inspiration Enlightenment Power Healing Peace Oneness Surrender Willingness Cheerfulness Magnetism Ascension	Pineal gland Thought Activates soul memories Center of the brain	Sixteen-second breath cycle Healing sound: AUM Healing musical note: E	Water Cauliflower White onions Spring onions Parsnip Pear Cabbage Garlic Coconut Cucumber water Lemon water **Chakra Recipe:** Blessed Water Pray over your water before drinking it. This energizes the water and infuses it with positive ions that activate the source of healing within and around us.	Rosemary Bergamot Amber Healing stones, gems, and crystals Diamond White tourmaline White jade Clear quartz

The Chakra Chart

Third Eye	Knowledge Intuition Command Divine Communication Understanding Completeness Intelligence Perceptions Certainty Revelation	Pituitary gland Above and between the eyes (with a stem at the back of the head) Hypothalamus Pineal gland	Eight-second breath cycle Healing sound: OM Healing musical note: G	Purple carrots Grapes Blackberries Wakame Nori Dulse Wheatgrass Sunflower greens Juice chakra: **High Priestess** 1 cup blackberries, 1 cup strawberries, 1/4 cabbage, 1 cucumber, handful of grapes, 1 apple, 1/4 lemon	Rose-geranium Violet Hyacinth White musk Healing stones, gems. and elements: Lapis lazuli Sapphire Pearl Amethyst Purple apatite Blue and white fluorite
Colors: indigo, turquoise, and mauve					

The Chakra Chart

Throat	Communication	Throat	Four-second	Blueberries	Hyacinth
	Clairvoyance		breath cycle	Blue corn	Patchouli
Colors:	Justice	Esophagus		Peas	White musk
blue, silver,	Purpose		Healing	Parsley	Lavender
turquoise	Voice	Larynx	sound: HAM	Cilantro	
	Speak and hear			Spirilina	
	Truth	Thyroid	Healing	Probiotics—	Healing
	Wisdom		note: G#	lacto	stones,
	Vibration				gems, and
					elements:
				Juice chakra:	
					Turquoise
				Blueberry	Sapphire
				Maca Root	Aquamarine
				Smoothie	Ether
					Akasha
				1 banana,	
				1/2 cup	
				hemp seed	
				milk, 1/2 cup	
				blueberries, 2	
				tablespoons	
				maca root	
				powder	

The Chakra Chart

Heart	Emotional power	Heart	Two-second breath cycle	Kale	Sandalwood
Spring green, rose, rose amethyst	Self-Expression Emotional balance Individuality Independence Joy Compassion Detachment Forgiveness	Lungs Thymus	Healing sound: YAM Healing note: D	Collards Aloe Cactus Pear Spinach Green apples Lime Leeks Avocado Wheatgrass Spirilina Young green coconut water and milk	Rose Honeysuckle Pine Healing stones, gems, and elements: Emerald Malachite Jade Green calcite Azurite Watermelon-Tourmaline
				Juice chakra: **Kale to the Queen** 2 kale leaves with stems, a big fistful of spinach, a handful of parsley, 1 cucumber, 1 lemon, 1 green apple	

The Chakra Chart

Solar Plexus Yellow, gold, rose	Consciousness Fire center The ability to act Understanding Discernment Self-esteem Relationship with self Maturation Logic Psychic intuition	Stomach Kidneys Enzyme production Metabolism Adrenals Digestive organs	One-second breath cycle Healing sound: RAM Healing note: A#	Lemon Squash Bananas Grapefruit Yellow bell peppers Millet Sesame seeds Sunflower seeds Juice chakra **Pineapple Orange Juice** 1/4 pineapple, 1 orange, 1/4 lemon, 2 carrots, 1 cucumber, 1/4 sweet potato	Rose Ylang ylang Bergamot Vetivert Healing stones, gems, and elements: Topaz Rose Quartz Yellow citrine Malachite

The Chakra Chart

Sacral	Reproduction	Abdominal	Half-second	Pumpkin	Rosemary
	Creativity	organs	breath cycle	Oranges	Rose
Orange,	Ancestral			Peppers	Geranium
amber	Intuition	Spleen	Healing	Flaxseeds	Amber
and gold	Desire		sound: VAM	Mangos	Musk
(nonmetallic)	Basic instincts	Reproductive		Carrots	
	and motives	organs	Healing	Butternut	Healing
	Sexual identity		note: C	squash	stones,
	Sensory	Fertility			gems, and
	Pleasure				elements:
	Relationships	Pancreas			
	Transformation			Juice chakra:	Topaz
		Intestines			Citrine
				WooTango	Amber
		Lymphatic		**Mango**	Aventurine
		system		**Tonic**	Moonstone
					Copper
				1 mango,	Jupiter
				1/2 lemon,	
				1 orange, 2	
				carrots, 1/2	
				cucumber	

The Chakra Chart

Root	Stability Survival	Perineum	Quarter-second	Beets Cherries	**Healing oils:**
Red, mauve, brown	Passion Anchored	Bowels	breath cycle	Pomegranates Cranberries	Lavender Cedarwood
	Right to have Self-Preservation	Legs	Healing sound: LAM	Red potatoes Grapefruit Red bell	Patchouli Hyacinth
	Rootedness Materialism Addiction Renewal		Healing note: A	peppers Peppers Chilies Red kidney beans	Healing stones, gems, and elements:
				Chia seeds Red delicious apples Flaxseeds Bartlett pear	Onyx Garnet Smoky quartz Ruby Agate
				Juice chakra:	Bloodstone Tiger's eye
				Cranberry Apple Juice	
				1 cup cranberries, 2 apples, 1/4 beet, 1 cucumber, 1/2 lemon	

A Beginners Guide to Chakra Balancing

In order for life force energy to flow unobstructed throughout your body, each chakra needs to be open and in balance with the others; this prevents disease and promotes well-being. Chakras can have too little energy or too much energy. Each state will create various imbalances that can affect mind and body. Balancing your chakras will release any stagnant energy and allow more energy to flow in. This will have a powerful effect within you and will reflect your outer experience of life!

There are many techniques you can use to bring your chakras into alignment; the general term for these techniques is chakra balancing. Because of the interconnection of the chakra system, balancing each chakra will affect the chakras on either side of it. What follows is a simple guide to balancing your chakras. You can do this by yourself or ask a partner to do it for you.

Preparation

1. Lie down comfortably on your back.
2. Clear any excess energy on your hands by shaking them.
3. When working on each chakra, picture it in perfect health.
4. Begin at the root chakra: place your hands a few inches above the body, palms facing down toward the chakra.

Cleansing

1. Keeping your hands the same distance from your body, slowly circle them counterclockwise (for one minute).
2. Finish this direction and shake your hands again to brush off excess energy (this has now cleansed your chakra).

Balancing

1. Now we want to balance it, and to do so we do the same as before but circling clockwise (for one minute).
2. Shake hands well upon completion.

Repetition

Continue these steps for each chakra, first cleansing it and then balancing it. It's as simple as that.

When you have worked with each chakra, simply rest and relax for a few moments while your body rebalances!

Keeping your chakras in vibrant health is a powerful addition to your well-being routine. Imagine them looking beautiful and radiant, sending energy with the power of your thoughts and attention. Mentally glancing up and down your body, checking in with your chakras and sharing some love can be done in under a minute and will ensure you get the maximum vitality from your life force energy.

Healing Affirmations for the Chakra

1. Be still and know.
2. Every hand that touches my hair is a healing hand.
3. Relaxation is the cure.
4. I am no longer in bondage to the past or future. Here now, all is well.
5. I'm always in the right place at the right time.
6. When I juice, I clear every doubt, every fear, every regret and perceived limitation.
7. I experience and express joy in everything I do.
8. I surround everything with love, every thought, every experience, every encounter, everything.
9. I am a love magnet. I attract only good into my life.

10. I am a money magnet. I am financially well, free, and unlimited.
11. Every thought is a prayer.
12. I forgive everyone for everything, with ease, grace, and cocoa butter.
13. With each inhale and exhale, I breathe love into everything and everyone.
14. I radiate peace.
15. I accept all of myself.
16. I allow Spirit to order every step in my life. I am divinely guided.
17. I never complain about the darkness, because I know I am the light.
18. I hold myself in the energy of love and acceptance at all times.
19. I see myself in all my glory.
20. My fro brings love to the world.
21. Be yourself.
22. I trust myself.
23. I can feel bad and recover.
24. There are angels all around me.
25. No matter where I am in the universe, I am safe.
26. I know myself.
27. I accept all of my intuitive gifts and use them with ease, while having fun in the process.
28. I appreciate myself.
29. I honor myself.
30. Om.
31. I honor my body.
32. I appreciate everyone who enters my life and experience.
33. I easily grow my medicine with ease and grace.
34. Harmony is at the core of all of my relationships.
35. Ashe.
36. Thank you.
37. And so it is.
38. I am who I've been waiting on.
39. I always get what I expect, so I expect only good.
40. As I heal, everyone I am connected to heals; everyone who thinks about me, remembers me, touches me, and sees me heals.

Spiritual Health and Well-Being Recipes

Bless This Kitchen

Everything you need is in the kitchen. You store your ingredients here, make them in this space, and care for yourself, your family, and friends from this epicenter of the earth.

The kitchen has its own affirmations and should be a place that brings you joy each time you enter and exit. Practice the affirmations and mindfulness activities below. Don't be surprised if you're inspired to create your own.

Affirmations

My laughter improves digestion.
I make joyful foods with ease here in my nourishment center.
Every appliance I touch energizes me with love.
Delicious abundance fills every inch of this kitchen.

Kitchen Mindfulness

Chant your favorite mantra while cooking.
Infuse good energy into your kitchen by meditating there once a week.
Each time you open the refrigerator, say a prayer.

Scalp Meditation

1. Massage love into your scalp.
2. Gently place your fingertips on your scalp and repeat silently, "I am that I am," as you massage each section.
3. Start from the back and work your way up to the front.

Hair Shedding

A former (or current) belief in deficiency, failure; feeling not good enough or that nobody cares; holding back; take a leap of faith; it's safe outside your comfort zone.

Not trusting your intuition, taking a passive approach to life.

Hair loss—release; out of balance with giving and receiving; rebirth, rejuvenation; ruminating over the past, present, or future.

I let each moment unfold with ease.

Treatment: reframe, rethink, rework—energize.

The biggest challenge most hair wearers want to prevent, or at least improve in some way.

Relaxing Tub Tea Recipe

Any method of focused concentration, practiced for a minimum of ten minutes, elicits the relaxation response. The relaxation response is the natural antidote to our mind and body's natural response to fear and anger (also referred to as the stress response—fight or flight). It's also an effective practice for relaxing the scalp and releasing constriction of the hair follicle.

The relaxation response also reverses the aging process, improves health, lowers blood pressure, helps relieve morning sickness, and reduces the symptoms of depression and anxiety. Make this relaxing tub tea and practice this powerful relaxation technique.

Place yourself in a state of peace and boost your spiritual health with this form of botanical therapy! This relaxing tub tea recipe is made with body-nourishing flowers, a lemony, light, uplifting essential oil, and the sweetest, most powerful, ingredient of all—you!

Simply get in and soak in the greatness (for about twenty minutes). Let any problem, tension, condition, energy, pattern, thought, pain, or state of consciousness that you would like to release go down the drain.

You Will Need:

- jumbo heat-and-seal tea bags
- an iron
- spoon
- fresh or dried flowers
- airtight plastic container, mason jar, or Ziploc bag

Ingredients

2 tablespoons lavender buds
2 tablespoons chamomile buds
1 tablespoon calendula flower
1 tablespoon hibiscus flower
5 to 10 drops lemon essential oil

Instructions

Add 1 to 2 tablespoons of dried flowers to your bags. You may find it easier to combine all of your ingredients in one bowl and then spoon out what you need. As long as you get everything into the bag and ready to seal, it's all good!

When I first tried to seal my tub teas, my iron wasn't hot enough. The directions said to keep the heat very low. This didn't work for me, and I typically use a high setting for a few seconds. Start with your iron on medium-high and go up from there.

That's it!

Add your tea to the bath. Your water may turn a slight tea color. Add bath oils if you are prone to dry skin. I like to add an essential-oil-infused safflower oil to the water (about 1 tablespoon).

To keep your tub teas fresh, store them in a mason jar, airtight container, or Ziploc bag.

Botanical Spotlight (and Spiritual Blessings)

Lavender

1. Lavender buds contain the pure, fragrant oil extracts that scent every lavender essential oil.
2. Lavender will also balance your skin's natural moisture levels and relieve a headache.
3. Often represents the spiritual principles of love, purity, and new beginnings. The color of royalty, lavender carries a majestic, lavishly abundant energy that is calming to the mind, heart, and body.
4. Although used as an insomnia cure, lavender has been clinically found to relieve stress, promote hair growth, relieve pain after surgery, eliminate insomnia, and make any tub tea a spa-level treatment.

Calendula Flower

1. Calendula flower is a powerful medicinal plant that speeds the healing of skin irritation, bruises, and burns.
2. It moisturizes dry skin and increases skins elasticity and firmness.
3. It is gentle enough for infants and children; used in creams, lotions, as fragrance, and in foods.
4. Elicits feelings of compassion and strengthens the spiritual principle of discernment.

Chamomile Flower

1. Promotes general relaxation and soothes the skin.
2. Strengthens intuition and helps us clarify and implement spiritual wisdom.
3. Heals dry skin; gets rid of dandruff.
4. Great for centering nervous energy.
5. Facilitates balance and emotional wellness.
6. The presence of this flower in your environment helps you become more forgiving of yourself and others.

Hibiscus Flower

1. In addition to stimulating hair growth, it is a natural source of alpha hydroxy acids, which are necessary for healthy, fresh, glowing skin.
2. Hibiscus naturally and gently exfoliates the skin, leaving behind soft, supple, well-nourished goodness.
3. It's super calming to the digestive and nervous systems. It soothes and cools nerve endings and balances all chakras.
4. Helps balance the reproductive system and boosts creativity.
5. Strengthens the spiritual principles of abundance, acknowledgment, and love.

Add more lavishly relaxing extras like:

Epsom salts
dead sea salts (don't use if you have high blood pressure)
essential oils (your favorite, or try something new!)

Chapter 16

The 21-Day Relaxation Diet

"We are all chemists in the laboratory of the Infinite. What, then, shall we create?"
Ernest Holmes, 365 Science of Mind

The Relaxation Diet is a 21-day self-management program designed to reduce stress and improve the health of your hair. This program combines the most effective, evidence-based treatments in health psychology, behavioral nutrition, and spirituality. Each day you are presented with a relaxation technique to practice. You'll also have a Juice Recipe of the Day, and mental vitamins (affirmations, quotes) to give your mind and body little boosts throughout the day.

The 21-Day Relaxation Diet is a based on an online and face-to-face self-management program I developed in 2006 called, LivingSMART (Stress Management & Relaxation Training). This program was created to help prevent and reduce postpartum stress, anxiety, and depression in new mothers. The diet that follows is a shortened version of the program that can be practiced in less than 20 minutes a day. It is a repeatable system designed to help you:

* prevent and reduce stress
* promote wellness
* and relax!

Let's get started!

To start the diet, let's assess where you are and establish your baseline scores (starting point:). We'll use these assessments to measure your results again at the end of the diet.

Pre-Diet Assessments

* The Perceived Stress Scale (PSS)
  http://www.psy.cmu.edu/~scohen/PSS.html

  For more about the PSS, visit Dr. Sheldon Cohen at Carnegie Mellon University: http://www.psy.cmu.edu/~scohen/

* Authentic Happiness Inventory, University of Pennsylvania
  https://www.authentichappiness.sas.upenn.edu

Day 1

Be Still and Know

Day 1 is the best. Our energy is high, we've completed the first steps (celebrate with some cool dance moves), and now we're in it to win it!

Today, set an intention for what you'd like to experience during this diet. Inhale deeply through your nose and out through your mouth to clear your mind.

Think about where you'd like to be at the end of the 21-days. *What do you want to be doing, and who do you want to be doing it with?* More importantly, *how's your hair?*

Have fun with it, think bigger than usual, and write your answers to the following three statements:

- *It is my intention…*
- *At the end of this diet…*
- *The one thing I'd love the most:*

Juice of the Day | Morning Green Juice

I know what you might be thinking … *Is that broccoli … stem?*

If you're nervous or if your taste buds revolt (this goes for any juice you make), you can always add another apple to sweeten.

Another option is to sweeten with stevia drops (no sugar, natural, and won't raise your blood sugar). They come in several different flavors and are extremely sweet. One drop is enough for several quarts of juice. Use it sparingly.

I use this type of stevia extract because it tastes good and it's easy to find at my local grocer.

Shop around for some in your area. Lemon drop is my favorite.

My Morning Green Juice

The Base

- kale leaves and stem
- a fistful of spinach
- 1/2 lemon
- cucumber

Add Natural Sweetness

- apple
- orange

Instructions

1. Wash and prep all ingredients.
2. Juice all ingredients.

Relaxation Activity: Practice Mindfulness for 10 Minutes.

Start by closing your eyes right where you are. Bring your shoulders up to your ears and squeeze gently. Lower your hands to your sides or place them in your lap and bring your attention to your breathing.

Don't change anything. Just be aware of the tempo, flow, and fullness of your breath.

Each time you breathe, you take in air from the four corners of the earth, the ocean, and etheric realm.

Breathe in whatever it is you feel you could use most in this moment. Breathe in joy; exhale joy. Breathe in peace; exhale peace.

Be still and know all is well.

Once you're complete with the meditation, wiggle your toes and your fingers. Slowly open your eyes.

Write about your experience and resume your awesome activities.

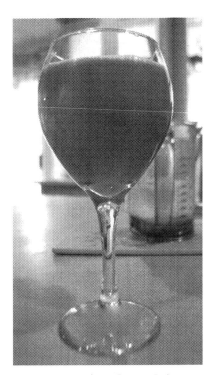

My Morning Green Juice

Day 2
Work The Root

Review the chakra chart on pages 198 - 204. Today, we'll explore the root chakra, which represents our connection to the earth, survival, and how anchored we are to the Inner Source.

Our sense of safety and security in the midst of transition is managed by the root. Our ability to heal our physical body begins and rests with this primary chakra. It helps us manage how we communicate and touch the world.

It's important to become aware of the energy, thoughts, colors, experiences, fragrances, and healing foods of all of the chakras.

Let's begin with the root, earth angel!

The Root Chakra

The color of the root chakra is a deep, almost crimson red. If you have red in your wardrobe, wear some today. If you don't have any red, see yourself surrounded by this energizing color.

Quick, try not to notice the red in the room where you are …

See what I'm talking about? It's now hard not to see the red that's all around you. The color red represents love, strength, good energy, courage, survival, and feeling connected to life and anchored to our soul.

Try this exercise focusing on everything good in your life. If you can't think of anything, focus on your heart beating, or being able to breathe on your own, your hands, being able to think and be and move—any and everything good that comes to mind. See yourself surrounded by good energy, good food, good people, and good health. Anytime you use the word good, you are also saying God. Wrap yourself in this sacred God energy.

The root chakra represents our connectedness to life, our ability to care for ourselves, our sense of safety and security, and the ability to comfort ourselves in times of transition.

Characteristics of the Root:

- self-centeredness
- right to have
- a desire for love and acceptance
- patience
- passion for living
- addiction
- materialism
- survival

When your mind and body are in balance, you are more likely to experience and express the higher energy states of the root: a passion for living, energized and looking forward to each day, knowing your safety and security is guaranteed and nonending, and being patient. An out-of-balance root chakra may trigger feelings and thoughts of being disconnected or alone, a tendency to think and focus on perceived threats to your survival, an increase in addictive behaviors, and an out of control appetite for material things.

Everyone gets out of balance from time to time. If you're not sure whether or not your root is having an out-of-balance experience, I've got you covered! Today's recipes will cleanse and detox old ideas, ways of being, and secret regrets from your system. I'll also introduce you to the chakra chart. Any mental or emotional issue that blesses your life can be resolved with the chakra. Read through the chart at least one time before focusing on the root chakra. We'll be working with this chart throughout the diet, so take baby steps.

A little healing goes a long way!

Juice Recipe of the Day | Cranberry Apple Juice

Heal, balance, and anchor the energy of your root chakra today with cranberry apple juice:

Ingredients

1 cup cranberries
2 apples
1/4 beet
1 cucumber
1/2 lemon

Instructions

1. Wash and prep all ingredients.
2. Juice all ingredients.

Relaxation Activity

Ground the energy in your chakra. Visit the meditation studio at EricaKKing.com/day-four and listen to the chakra meditation.

Write about your meditation experience. Notice any sensations, revelations, or insights you were not aware of before.

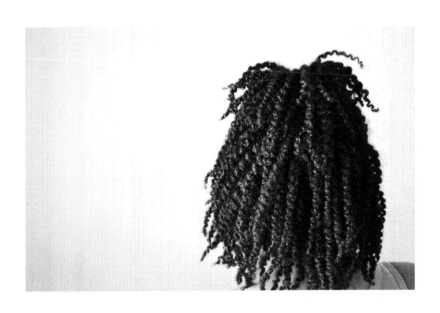

The Sacral Chakra

Review the chakra chart on pages 198 - 204. Today, we'll explore the sacral chakra, which represents creativity, fertility, and relationships.

Having a problem getting started or moving forward? Check the energy of your sacral chakra. Having problems with conception, vaginal who knows what, migraines, or allergies?

Bring more orange into your life and work with this chakra.

All of your basic instincts and ancestral memories live in the sacral chakra. The inner knowingness you were born with, and your ability to feel in your mind, body, and experience are all here in the sacral.

The sacral chakra holds our ancestral memories, feelings, symbols, and secrets. Our sensual awareness and sexual identity live in this chakra, along with our sense of accomplishment, and the ability to bring our desires to life.

The Color Orange

The sacral chakra is a bright, rich orange color that reminds you of a sweet, plump orange. The color orange evokes feelings of peace and even a bit of euphoria. An out-of-balance sacral can have you feeling like a complete failure. You'll have a million reasons why this is, but none of them will be accurate. It's just a feeling. Repeat the scriptural affirmation: And this too shall pass, and keep it moving.

If you focus on this feeling, it can stick around and lead to feelings of hostility and a resistance to seemingly everything,

What you resist, persists.

What persists, can lead to reproductive challenges and an inability to move forward on your ideas and goals.

Characteristics of an Out-of-Balance Sacral:

1. An out of balance sacral can cause you to be overly critical and to feel you are being overly criticized.
2. An increase in gossiping, bullying or being bullied
3. An inability to distinguish between right and wrong, negative and positive feelings.
4. An out of balance sacral blocks creativity which can show up as fibroids, growths, cysts, and tumors in and around the uterus.

When your mind and body are in balance, you are more likely to experience and express the higher energy states of the sacral chakra: feeling alive, clear, confident, and accountable.

Just like with our rowdy root chakra, everyone gets out of balance from time to time. If you're not sure whether or not your sacral is having an out-of-balance experience, I've got you covered!

Today's Sacral Balancing Affirmations:

WIth each breath I break all ancestral curses.

My pleasure pleases God.

I can feel bad and recover.

Other Sacral Characteristics:

- *Sexual health, sexual identity.*
- *This chakra controls all of your reproductive organs.*
- *The ability to give and receive pleasure (in all things).*
- *Sensory alignment and awareness.*
- *self-control*
- *right to feel*
- *the ability to give and receive pleasure*

- *basic instincts*
- *body awareness, acceptance*
- *clear boundaries*
- *our sense of accomplishment*
- *spontaneity*

An out-of-balance sacral chakra may increase feelings and experiences of hostility, complete failure, criticism, or gossip. Blocked, dormant creativity in the organs that govern this chakra can show up as fibroids, cysts, and growths in and around the uterus.

Try This:

Wrap yourself in an orange blanket, breathe in the color orange, and tune into the area right underneath your belly button … or drink the juice and go to sleep! If you're interested in energy medicine, try my chakra-purifying meditation below.

Remember: be the orange!

Juice Recipe of the Day | WooTango Mango

Ingredients

1 mango
1/2 lemon
1 orange
2 carrots
1/2 cucumber

Instructions

1. Cleanse and prep your ingredients.
2. Run them through the juicer in the order presented.
3. Pour them in your glass or cup and enjoy!

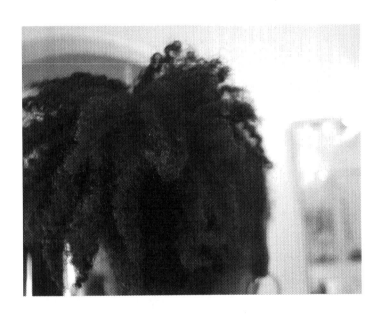

Day 4
Make Your Own Hair Cleanser

Today's Diet: make one of the **Six All-Natural Cleansers for Beautiful, Natural Hair:**

1. *Soap Nut Foam Clarifying Shampoo*
2. *Erica's Honey-Love Clay Wash*
3. *Chelating Cactus Syrup*
4. *Cherry Club Soda*
5. *Lavishly Natural's Herbal Shampoo*
6. *Super Bowl Clay Wash*

Juice Recipe of the Day | Pineapple Ginger

This is a wonderful morning and midday juice. Pineapple is easily digested by your system, which means your body can convert it to superpower energy and a more peaceful state of mind. Packed with vitamins and minerals, pineapple also has:

- vitamins A, B1, B2, B3, B6, B12, C, D, E, K
- boron
- calcium
- chloride
- chromium
- copper
- fluoride
- iodine
- iron
- magnesium
- manganese
- molybdenum
- phosphorus
- potassium
- selenium
- sodium
- zinc

Pineapples are one of the few fruits you can buy that doesn't have to be organic. Its tough skin protects its vitamin and mineral goodness. It's the perfect fruit to eat when you're feeling blue. It's rich in B vitamins, which help you feel good, awaken new and dormant nerve endings in the body, and soothe an anxious thought system. Raw pineapple juice is a wonderful chaser to have or mix with your weekly wheatgrass shots (at least two ounces)!

Especially if you're like me and need a little something to enjoy it!

Pineapples also:

1. *Improve memory*
2. *Are calming to your system*
3. *Easily digestible and highly nutritious*
4. *Reduces inflammation of the digestive tract, ulcers, and poor circulation*
5. *Detoxifying*
6. *Boosts clarity*
7. *Inspires creativity*

Pineapple Ginger Recipe

1/2 or 1 whole pineapple
1 big fistful of kale
2 cucumbers
1 lemon
optional: 1/4 inch of ginger

1. Cleanse, peel, and prepare all fruit and vegetables.
2. Add ingredients to your juicer or blender.
3. Drink like your life depends on it!

Affirmation:

I forgive everyone for everything with ease, grace, and cocoa butter.

Milk Bath for the Inner Goddess

There is no need to go to India or anywhere else to find peace. You will find that
deep place of silence right in your room, your garden or even your bathtub.
—Elizabeth Kubler-Ross

Hello, Love!

It's been five days of health, wholeness, and perfection, and that's just you waking up in the morning!

Your body now knows it is not in control and may be feeling some type of way about it. If you have any aches or pains, tense places, or tired joints, today's recipe will cure them all. It is important to take warm baths during the relaxation diet, as water has its own unique healing properties.

Today's Diet: Take a skin healing milk bath!

Milk and Honey Bath Recipe

Ingredients:

1/4 cup warm honey
1 gallon whole milk (go crazy and get organic)
1/2 teaspoon vanilla extract (optional for fragrance)
1/4 cup fresh or dried chamomile, rose, or lavender flowers

Instructions

1. Heat 1 cup of milk on medium heat. Add honey and reduce heat to low. Simmer until honey is mixed in completely.
2. Run a hot bath.

3. Add this cup of milk and remaining gallon to your bath. If it's too hot, you don't have to enter right away (it's never supposed to be painful).
4. Add your fresh flowers to the bath water and let sit for at least 10 minutes.
5. Enter, relax, and let the milk and honey do all the work.

This skin-softening milk bath is wonderful with any type of milk. You can glam it up, make it way more decadent if you like. Some fasters use goat milk, while others have found success with powdered milk. For powdered milk recipes, use four big tablespoons of organic powdered milk.

Bath Exercise:

1. *Soak for a minimum of twenty minutes.*
2. *Before leaving the tub, visualize any challenge, problem, illness, or blockage leaving your mind and body and flowing down the drain, forever washed away.*

After your bath, use one of the:

The Seven Healing Butters of the Chakra

Each chakra has its own healing butter. These butters help to open, balance, and recalibrate it's specific chaka. As you work it into your hair and skin, you are purifying and grounding the chakra's healing energy within you and around you.

Crown
Raw Shea Butter

Third Eye
Kokum Butter

Throat
Illipe Butter

Heart
Avocado Butter

Solar Plexus
Cupuacu Butter

Sacral
Mango Butter

Root
Cocoa Butter

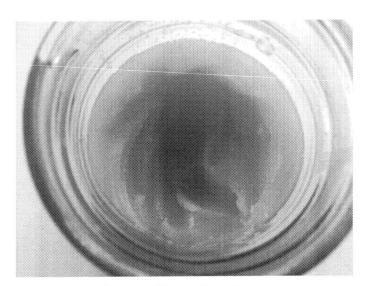

Cupuacu Mango Shea Butter

Skin-lovin' alternatives for cow's milk in this bath:

- *Goat's milk has the same pH as human skin and is quite effective for attaining smoother skin.*
- *Oat milk contains oat grain, which is super for sensitive skin because it soothes as it moisturizes.*
- *Rice milk is also terrific for hydrating the skin and promoting healthy new cells.*

Day 6
The Power Chakra

Today's Diet: Make the healing oil recipe from page 97. Use it as an all-over-body oil to balance your solar plexus.

We have moved the energy and balanced our first two chakra — the root and sacral chakras. Today, we'll going to unleash the power of our solar plexus which is located at the base of the sternum. It's known by it's yellow color and represents our basic will, our purpose, consciousness, who we are, and what we can do.

Review the chakra chart on pages 198 - 204. Select one healing treatment, sound, or stone for the solar plexus. If you don't have the actual item, a picture, photo or video of it will work the same way. Strengthen your imagery and visualization skills by seeing, feeling or imaging one of the healing stones for this chakra (topaz, rose, and quartz are three of them).

The Fire Center

The solar plexus is our fire center and when it's in balance, there's no-thing we cannot do. This is the chakra of independence, respect for differences and acknowledging the truth. That strength you didn't know you had, the peace that surpasses all understanding, lives in this chakra.

It's so powerful it has it's own breathing exercise often referred to in yoga as Pranayama Breath, or *Breath of Fire*. This rapid breathing exercise can dissolve the thickest grief, the worst anger, and the most isolating sadness. An out-of-balance solar plexus may show up as experiences that trigger insecurity, inferiority, shame, obsession or control.

Although challenging at times, these experiences allow us to effectively negotiate our internal and external conflicts so that anger and fear don't multiply.

Characteristics of the Solar Plexus

- *right ideas, right action, right results*
- *manages metabolism, the stomach and digestion, kidneys, and adrenal glands*
- *spiritual principle: acceptance, discernment*
- *stillness, silence & peace*
- *expanding limits*
- *confidence*
- *power - the ability to mold, shape into existence*
- *a conscious realization that "I am loved by God"*

Something else to know about the solar plexus, if you're experiencing lot's of loss in your life — loss of hair, friends, property, love, or jobs go yellow everything! When you experience any type of loss, it's a signal that something is off or out of balance. Place fresh yellow flowers around your home: dandelions, sunflowers, yellow lillies (which bring financial blessings), yellow roses, tulips. Use fresh lemons to decorate your space and add a fresh splash of yellow to the room.

Faith and belief are the channels of power.

One of the best things to do do balance, boost, and re-activate your solar plexus is to fast!

I know what you're thinking, you're not into starvation. Neither am I. Fasting for a few hours or for 30 days requires the same thing — great recipes! There's only so much kale you can down before you really feel like you'll eat the juicer, especially if it's covered in barbeque sauce.

The key to a good fast is to never get hungry. Sounds a little backwards right, because we're not eating and all, but let me show you what I mean.

Fast-A-Palooza

When I run Fast-A-Palooza (a 30-Day Online Juice Fast), I get hundreds of questions. Some people are fasting for a few hours, a few days, a week, a full month or even longer. Our goal is to support each other during the fast with positive energy, tips, ad tools. It's a blast! During this live fast, hundreds of questions come in each week. One of the most common is, *what do I do when I'm tired of juicing?*

Alicia M. from DC writes:

"I'm tired of juice already. I'm going to turn into spinach. I'm not hungry all the time but I do miss food when my boyfriend is eating. Any tips?"

Absolutely, I've got the perfect recipes for that!

Create "meals" even while fasting.

Include soups (if homemade, make them liquid consistency), pureed veggies, and frozen treats during your fast. You don't have to drink the same things all the time, unless you like a particular drink or if you live next to a kale farm (my dream). I buy lots of whatever is in season and then grab a few favorites.

I've included "fast" meals below. Be creative and don't forget to drink lost of water. Some fasters like to drink up to a gallon a day. It's up to you! Water will keep you hydrated and flushed with aqua awesomeness. I drink about two liters or more throughout the day. How about you?

Fast Meals

Breakfast

Hot water with lemon: wakes up the body in a gentle way.

Morning juice: something with kale and cucumber. Try Green Goddess, My Morning Green Juice, or Green Buddha. Start the day green!

2 ounces home-grown wheatgrass

Lunch

Pureed soup, liquid consistency. You can also warm vegetable broth (or make your own) and sip it; it will be the best "soup" you've ever had. If you have a hand blender, it's excellent for a quick puree.

Dinner

Water

Pureed Vegetable Soup

Dessert

Green Tea Smoothie

1 1/2 cup hemp seed milk
1/2 peeled peach (if using frozen peaches, use 1/2 cup)
1/2 teaspoon vanilla
1 teaspoon matcha green tea
1./2 teaspoon raw agave syrup
a handful of ice

Instructions

1. Add all of the ingredients to a high speed blender.
2. Blend for up to 1 minute or until smooth.
3. Pour into your favorite glass and enjoy!

Note

I use Encha's Ceremonial Grade Matcha Green Tea for this recipe. Fresh matcha green tea is bright green in color. When shopping for your perfect tea, make sure to let your eyes do the choosing. If it looks dull or like baby poop, steer clear! For Encha's matcha goodness, visit them at Encha.com.

Relaxation Activity: Observing the Breath (OTB)

Observing the breath is the most powerful form of meditation.

Simply observing your breathing is the meditation. You may also use breathing techniques to:

- center yourself before a meditation
- instantly relieve stress or anxiety
- a way to end any activity and relaxation session

Throughout the day, take time to notice the texture of the air you breathe:[52]

Is it heavy?
Is it light?
Is it course?
Is it smooth?
Is it moist?
Is it dry?

Notice the air as it passes through, over, within, and around your:

- nostrils
- lips
- mouth
- throat
- lungs

With a deep, detoxing breath (breathe in through the nose, out through the mouth), tune in to the muscles of the chest, the belly (abdomen), the shoulders, and diaphragm (below the breast bone).

Place your hands over the muscles and notice how they feel:

- relaxed
- tensed
- solid
- loose

Be aware of any sensations in the body, limbs, and scalp.

Diet Bonus | Healing Herbs, Oils, and Essentials

Essential Oils for Hair Growth, Mental Balance, and Acceptance: rosemary, basil, thyme, ylang ylang, peppermint

Botanicals for Hair Growth, Mental Relaxation, and Spontaneous Happiness: maca root, fenugreek seeds, slippery elm powder

Recipes for Healing, Cleansing, Detoxification, and Mega Hair Growth:

Bentonite Clay Wash: 1 cup bentonite clay, 2 cups apple cider vinegar, 2 tablespoons marshmallow root powder, 2 tablespoons honey, 2 tablespoons castor oil (or coconut oil), 2 tablespoons shea butter.

Dandelion Hair Tea: 1 tablespoon (or 1 tea bag) dandelion root, 2 tablespoons flaxseeds, 2 1/2 cups water, 5 drops lemon essential oil (or 1 teaspoon of lemon juice) 1 tablespoon honey, optional—1 to 2 teaspoons apple cider vinegar

Catnip Hair Tea: 2 tablespoons catnip, 2 cups hot water, 6 drops lavender essential oil

Juice Recipes for Soul Renewal and Perfect Health:

High Priestess: 1 cup blackberries, 1 cup strawberries, 1/4 cabbage, 1 cucumber, handful of grapes, 1 apple, 1/4 lemon

Kale to the Queen: 2 kale leaves with stems, a big fistful of spinach, a handful of parsley, 1 cucumber, 1 lemon, 1 green apple

Red Goddess: 1 pear, 1/4 lemon, 2 carrots, 1/2 beet, a handful of beet greens, a handful of spinach, 1 cucumber

Vegetables for Spiritual Wellness: kale, spinach, cucumber, carrots, beets, red, purple, and green cabbage, broccoli, cauliflower, garlic, onion, red, yellow, orange bell peppers

Day 7
Mental Fitness

Green juices are popular, but it's the rainbow of colors that keeps you healthy and awesome! Red Goddess is a blend of beetroot, beet greens, spinach, and cucumber.

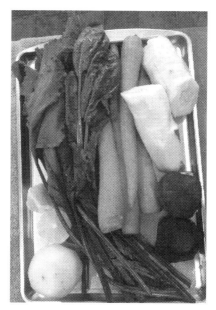

Red Goddess Ingredients

Mental Fitness: Know Thyself

Acknowledgment, as a spiritual practice, is a luscious process of recognition. It does not justify or explain. It never requires a defense. Acknowledgement is always the first step in healing.

The Knowing Practice

Knowing yourself is really the practice of acknowledgment. When you know yourself, you no longer repeat the same mistakes over and over again. You now know what to do and you get busy doing it!

You know how and when to get still. You trust your ability to hear and discern the divine guidance you receive. You also know in your curls that right here, right now, all is perfect, whole, and complete. You lack no-thing. Know you'll be successful in all that you are and all that you do. Rest in this energy and move in the direction of the guidance you receive.

The Non-Judgment Two-Step

Did you know that when you are not judging yourself (criticizing, berating, chastising, shoulda, woulda, coulda-ing yourself), your mind will naturally clear? Mental confusion disappears, and new ideas rush forth.

Relaxation occurs in mind, body, and soul anytime judgment (conflicting thought) is absent. It's the natural cleanser that enhances confidence and faith in yourself.

1. *Call a thing a thing. Recognize any thing for what it is. Own it and embrace it without criticism.*
2. *Acknowledgment precedes all forward movement in life; it does not mean that you know what to do.*

Declare:

"Everything I need to know is given to me, provided for me, told to me, delivered to me right when I need to know it, in the right way, at the right time, with the right people, in the right energy. I am always in the right place at the right time."

Mental Vitamins: Try These Cognitive-Behavioral Statements for Healing Stress

I accept the natural rhythms and cycles of life with ease and grace.

Ancient wisdom grows within each strand of my hair. I always know what I need to know, when I need to know it.

I am prospered by every change that flows into my life.

My healing comes from within.

Juice Recipe of the Day | Red Goddess

1 pear
1/4 lemon
2 carrots
1/2 beet
handful of beet greens
handful of spinach
1 cucumber

Instructions

1. Wash, prep, and peel your ingredients.
2. Run them through your juicer in the order listed.

Options:

Add stevia or your sweetener of choice if needed.
Also tastes awesome over ice!

Relaxation Activity

Write the following statement in your journal, on a note card, or Post-It note. Say it out loud. Repeat this mantra anytime you feel out of balance or upset. It is an energetic dissolving agent.

"Nothing is broken and nothing needs to be fixed. When I dwell in this awareness, all my wounds are healed. Miracles happen."

Use this as your mantra throughout the day.

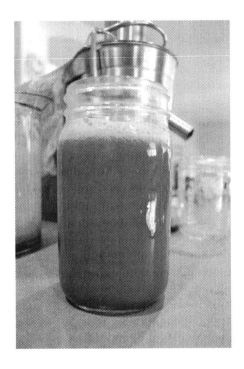

Day 8
Kale To The Queen

Today's affirmation: I am always supported by seen and unseen help.

Kale is my favorite veggie. Up to about a year ago, I would have put it in the collard-mustard green category, believing it must be cooked to be any good. WebMD[73] reports kale as having 134 percent of the daily value of vitamin C, 206 percent of vitamin A, and 689 percent of vitamin K. It should be called bodacious K! Not to be left out, it also has 9 percent of calcium.

Kale is abundantly filled with antioxidants like carotenoids and flavonoids that fight cancer and sulfur-containing phytonutrients that also help this veggie:

- lower cholesterol
- improve skin
- enhance eye health
- strengthen bones
- reduce the risk of heart disease

Thanks to Kris Carr and her book, Crazy Sexy Kitchen, I ventured into juicing this cruciferous vegetable from the mustard family (or brassica family for my foodies out there), which includes:

- broccoli
- turnips
- cabbage
- rutabaga
- cauliflower
- Chinese cabbage
- brussels sprouts
- kale
- collards
- mustard greens

There are several varieties of kale that are perfect for juicing (Italian and dinosaur are fun).

Watch me make this goodie in my <u>Kale to the Queen</u> video here: https://youtu.be/HeRf8b_PQeo.

Juice Recipe of the Day | Kale to the Queen

Ingredients:

5 kale leaves (or a big handful)
3 apples
4 carrots
3 oranges

1. Cleanse and prep your ingredients.
2. Naturally balance your heart chakra.
3. Juice and enjoy!

Relaxation Activity | Get to Know Your Heart Chakra

Review the chakra chart on page 201. The heart chakra governs the heart and lungs. When in balance, you have a strong sense of worthiness and self-confidence from all of the work you've done clearing the lower levels and your ability to complete and master whatever you set out to do.

A statement the heart chakra would say might begin with: You can tell I love myself …

You can tell I love myself by how I speak to myself and others.
You can tell I love myself by whom I surround myself with.
You can tell I love myself by what I eat.

Finish the following sentences:

You can tell I love myself when...
I know I am love, loving, loved, and lovable because...

An out-of-balance heart chakra will lead to challenges with emotional expression, individuality, and procrastination.

To strengthen and clear your heart chakra, add more of these foods to your meals:

- *kale*
- *collards*
- *aloe*
- *cactus*
- *pear*
- *spinach*
- *green apples*
- *lime*
- *leeks*
- *avocado*
- *wheatgrass*
- *Spirilina*
- *young green coconut water*

Day 9
Flower Therapy

Flower therapy is a how-to guide for adding real flower power to your life! When focused on through meditation, appreciating their natural beauty, or given as a gift to brighten someone's day, flower therapy can provide comfort and joy.

Defined as "a method of using different blossoms for specific needs and desires,"[106] naturopaths Robert Reeves and Doreen Virtue, authors of *Flower Therapy*, provide several different ways to use flower treatments, including:

- flower meditations
- prayers
- working with angels and fairies
- cutting and caring for flowers
- giving flowers to others
- chakra balancing
- how to pick wildflowers
- even how to care for wilted flowers

Flower Infusions

Since I make mostly all of my natural hair and skin-care products, I was particularly interested in the chapter on flower essences and infusions. I use organic roses and hibiscus flowers in my homemade clay wash, rinses, and bath salts. These along with flower extracts, powders, and essential oils have helped me with hair growth and healing my skin—get back, eczema.

In addition to extra softening, conditioning, and fabulousness, I learned that red roses:

- have motivating energy

- promote healing
- attract more love
- boost passion

Pink roses provide:

- comfort
- beauty
- self-confidence
- being content with yourself

When my husband filled our kitchen with a bouquet of fresh orange lilies and yellow daisies, I couldn't wait to go to the flower therapy chart to read the full list of each flower's personality, energetic properties, and message (after hugs and kisses of course).

Lily (Orange)

- good for calmness
- good for releasing excess baggage
- good for weight loss (Who knew?)

Daisy

- great for removing drama and stress
- great for relaxation
- great for self-care

What's also good about *Flower Therapy* is that each page is filled with vibrant colors. This was great for flowers I wasn't familiar with and for opening to a random page and enjoying a nice bouquet of hydrangea.

The flowers are beautiful, and if you don't have fresh flowers or prefer not to cut or remove them from their natural environment, a picture is just as effective!

Juice Recipe of the Day: Grapefruit Juice, Freshly Squeezed

1 whole grapefruit
1 plastic hand juicer

Instructions

1. Slice grapefruit in half.
2. Juice with a smile.
3. Makes about 12 ounces.

Grapefruit Juice Benefits

Grapefruit juice has many superpowers. It can cut the fat content of your meals, prevent sugar cravings, and naturally suppress your appetite.

It's also a superpower food for shaping and toning your belly-dancing abs, so say Neena and Veena Bidasha, belly-dancing twins and authors of *The Way of the Belly: 8 Essential Secrets of Beauty, Sensuality, Health, Happiness and Outrageous Fun*. Get your belly and hips ready … this book comes with a belly-dancing CD!

Relaxation Activity: Forgiveness Practice | Morning & Evening

Write thirty-five forgiveness statements now and again right before you go to bed.

At a loss for words? No worries!

You can use these to get you started.

1. I, (your first name), forgive myself fully and completely.
2. I forgive myself and everyone else for everything with ease and grace.

3. I forgive myself for judging myself as:
4. I forgive myself for judging others as …
5. I forgive (name of the person you find it hardest to forgive) for …

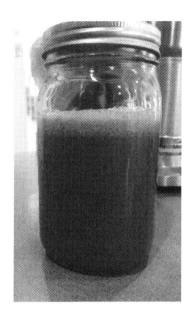

Day 10
Choose Your Signature Affirmation

Perhaps it's the eternal student in me, but I take notes on everything I read. I love reading, writing, and speaking affirmations (aka verbal meditations) so that they become planted and deeply rooted in the garden of my mind.

Affirmations are statements of truth that have a cognitive (what we think), behavioral (what we do), and emotional effect (how we feel). Think of them as powerful re-enforcers, dissolving agents, and insurance that you are the master of your mind, not mastered by your mind. Every thought carries its own energy, and so do affirmations.

They are the language of the soul! The best affirmations are the ones you write. Use these during the remaining days of the diet, or my favorite, while doing your hair!

Infuse good energy into each strand with each word and touch. "Every hand that touches my hair is a healing hand." Hair affirmations (mini cognitive-behavioral treatments) are equally as effective as our hair oils, butters, and yes, I'll say it … cactus gels!

Create your own affirmations or mantras. You probably have a few you use all the time. Review the list below. If your hair had a mantra, what would it be?

Select one below or create your own.

Forty Hair Affirmations for Health and Wellness

1. *Be still and know.*
2. *My heart pumps pure love all through my body.*
3. *Relaxation is the cure.*
4. *I am no longer in bondage to the past or future. Here now, all is well.*
5. *I'm always in the right place at the right time.*
6. *When I juice, I clear every doubt, every fear, every regret, and perceived limitation.*

7. *I experience and express joy in everything I do.*
8. *I surround everything with love, every thought, every experience, every encounter, every-thing.*
9. *I am a love magnet. I attract only good into my life.*
10. *I am a money magnet. I am financially well, free, and unlimited.*
11. *Every thought is a prayer.*
12. *I forgive everyone for everything, with ease, grace, and cocoa butter.*
13. *With each inhale and exhale, I breathe love into everything and everyone.*
14. *I radiate peace.*
15. *I accept all of myself.*
16. *I allow Spirit to order every step in my life. I am divinely guided.*
17. *I never complain about the darkness, because I know I am the light.*
18. *I hold myself in the energy of love and acceptance at all times.*
19. *I see myself in all my glory.*
20. *My fro brings love to the world.*
21. *Be yourself.*
22. *I trust myself.*
23. *I can feel bad and recover.*
24. *There are angels all around me.*
25. *No matter where I am in the universe, I am safe.*
26. *I know myself.*
27. *I accept all of my intuitive gifts and use them with ease while having fun in the process.*
28. *I appreciate myself.*
29. *I honor myself.*
30. *I am worthy.*
31. *I honor my body.*
32. *I appreciate everyone who enters my life and experience.*
33. *I easily grow my medicine with ease and grace.*
34. *Harmony is at the core of all of my relationships.*
35. *Amen.*
36. *Thank you.*
37. *And so it is.*
38. *I. Can. Do. This.*
39. *I am who I've been waiting on.*
40. *I always get what I expect, so I expect only good.*

My Signature Affirmation(s):

_____

_____

_____

_____

_____

_____

_____

_____

_____

Juice Recipe of the Day | Green Goddess

If there was an award for best green juice taste, this one would win! It tastes like a juicy punch with fruits and veggies that love being together. You can tell!

There are lots of Green Goddess recipes. If you juice long enough (over a day) you'll make one up of your own!

Here's mine …

Lavishly Natural's Green Goddess Recipe

1/2 pineapple
big fistful of kale
big fistful of spinach
1 cucumber
1 orange
1 mango
1 nectarine

Instructions

1. Smile as you cleanse and prepare your ingredients.
2. Juice them while doing a happy dance.
3. Pour her in your chilled glass and sip.

Relaxation Activity | Breathe

Sit for at least ten minutes in silence. No distractions. No phones, e-mails, texts, or tweets. Close your eyes, get comfy, and breathe. Don't change the rhythm of your breathing; just bring your awareness to it. If thoughts begin to flood your mind, inhale deeply and observe them. Let them go by as if you're watching them floating down a stream. Bring your attention back to the breath. This is a conscious act of letting go.

Diet Bonus: Breathing Meditation

Listen to Satori, my version of the Brilliant Body Scan. The body scan is a relaxation exercise that helps the body mental and emotional toxins from the joints, organs and tissues of the body. Plus, it sounds really cool. This relaxation exercise is approximately 18:21. Access it here: *EricaKKing. com/satori.*

Day 11
Who Am I?

*I am open and receptive to more good than I have ever experienced
before, than anyone has ever experienced before.*
—Michael Bernard Beckwith

Awareness

Awareness is "an internal process which transforms experience into wisdom, and confusion into clarity."[52] Bring awareness to any upset, challenge, or fear, and it will have no choice but to dissolve right then and there.

The key is to learn how to drop your defenses (beliefs, values, unnecessary competition, personal myths, excuses, justifications, the need to be right, rationales, and perceived limitations) so that you can stay in the flow of life. This will keep your heart, mind, and soul stay clear and open.

Awareness makes the unclear, clear.

It is mental and emotional recognition that a thing exists.[52] Awareness is what you take with you when whatever you are facing seems menacing, uncomfortable, or has a potential for any type of pain. It will always—*always*—lead you to the highest, best possible outcome for you and all others involved.

Today's activities are designed to boost and strengthen your awareness. We'll do this by working with the power chakra from Day 6: the solar plexus. If you have some yellow, wear it today. Put it in your space and keep it in your beautiful face! The color yellow facilitates a natural shift in how you feel and an even deeper experience of joy! It is the color of happiness as evident by the classic smiley face and smiley face emoji!

See Yourself

You become attuned to what's happening in your life moment by moment. This way you become aware of how you respond or react to life. You can prevent reactions by becoming aware of their triggers. This awareness gives way to a state of empowerment where you can make new choices and dissolve old patterns, pain, and wounds.

To practice seeing yourself, refer back to your chakra chart on day 2. Bring your awareness to the solar plexus.

The solar plexus is often referred to as your power center, your core. A balanced solar plexus is often yellow or gold. Your sense of purpose and the ability to discern the truth in all things is managed within this chakra.

Instructions

To practice seeing your divine self, answer the following questions. Capture the first thought that comes into your mind by recording. If you have a smartphone, use the voice memo. You'll want to play back your answers. Don't have a recorder? Tell three other people your answers. They may or may not be people you know.

Who am I?
What can I do?
What do I stand for?

Other characteristics of a healed solar plexus:

- a significant desire for all to be respected for their differences
- speeds the completion of small doable tasks
- where your life purpose lives (It was imprinted on your soul before you were born.)
- acknowledgment, awareness, and ability to tell the truth
- independence

- attuned psychic ability
- balanced internal and external conflict

Juice Recipe of the day | Pineapple Orange Juice

Pineapple Orange Juice balances, grounds, and clears the solar plexus.

Ingredients

1/2 pineapple
1 orange
1 peach
1 large carrot
2 fistfuls of kale
2 small cucumbers

Instructions

1. Cleanse and prep your ingredients.
2. Run them through the juicer in the order presented.

Optional:

Leave out the kale and add 1/4 inch of cabbage. To sweeten this juice naturally, add 1/4 inch ripe sweet potato and 1/4 cup of mango!

Cabbage reduces belly fat. It's full of fiber and calms the digestive system. It naturally detoxifies the body and lifts a low mood.

Identify Your Clairvoyance (Clear Vision)

You are already aware of your intuitive abilities. They've been passed down to us for centuries as each generation surveys and thrives in the era that it's in.

Just as there are different learning styles, we all have intuitive, psychic abilities. This means we pick up or key in to information that we otherwise have no way to access and know.

We're born with these skills much like we're born with the ability to nurse right after delivery. Without this innate ability, we could not receive the nourishment needed to grow.

The same is true for our clairvoyant gift and talents.

Clairvoyance is defined as:

> "The power of discerning objects not present to the senses but regarded as having objective reality [things we know exist independently of us]. Intuitive perception; clear vision; Everything that takes place in the world of manifestation first takes place in the realm of thought. If one is spiritually quickened to the measure that [she] can discern the thought movements, [she] can gain a foreknowledge of what is about to occur (Fillmore, 1997, p. 38)."

You can use clairvoyance to get mentally and emotionally unstuck, to let go of the past, and to change your health from the inside out, all without having any knowledge of how to do so. Clairvoyance presents in four different types. You were born with all four but may be stronger in one more than the others.

There are four primary types of clairvoyance[64] that we all have. They are:

Clairaudience *(clairaudient, clear hearing)* — receives messages, guidance, divine information, through sound, voice, music, hearing, listening; can come from outside or inside the mind

Clairsentience *(clairsentient, clear feeling)* — receives messages, guidance, and divine information through feelings, senses, emotions, smell, taste

Clairvoyance (clear seeing)—receives messages from all the senses and beyond the physical realm; messages can take the form of still images, miniature movies or dreams.

Claircognizance (claircognizant, clear knowing)—receive messages, guidance, and divine information through thought, ideas, pictures, images, revelations, symbols

What's Your Primary Clair?

To discover what your clairvoyant style is, read *Divine Guidance* by Doreen Virtue. It contains several exercises that will help you identify your divine communication style. She's also put together a brief Q&A to help you identify which clair may be strongest for you.

Take the test here:
https://hayhouseoz.wordpress.com/2011/02/03/whats-your-primary-clair-doreen-virtue/

Juice Recipe of the Day: Bluepeary Apple Juice

Strengthens the third eye chakra and boosts clairvoyance.

Ingredients

1/4 cup blueberries (fresh)
1 apple
1 pear
1 cucumber
3 kale leaves with stems

Instructions

1. Wash and peel the apple, pear, and cucumber. Rinse the blueberries and kale leaves.
2. Run ingredients through your juicer.
3. Drink within 15 minutes for maximum nutrient and vitamin absorption ... although anytime is a good time for green juice!

Day 13
Create A Personal Logo

When what you say, think, and feel is in harmony, you experience the peace that surpasses all understanding. To be yourself, you must have inner cooperation in the mental, spiritual, emotional, and physical areas of your life. Be willing to live beyond the limitations placed upon you by others and by yourself.

The Goddess Formerly Known As...

If you could only identify yourself as a symbol from this moment forward, what symbol would you be? Is there one that immediately comes to mind? Are there several symbols, shapes, or images that come to mind?

For today's diet, we're going to create a visual reminder of the great elements that make you unique and awesome! If you can't draw, no worries! Your personal logo comes from your soul. It's as special as a fingerprint. You are the only artist that can design it!

One more thing...

A personal logo should cause you to feel good each and every time you see it. If it doesn't, it can't work its magic! They're super simple to make and only require a little imagination.

To get started, gather the following items:

- paper
- construction paper (all colors)
- crayons
- markers
- glitter of any type
- scissors
- tape
- glue sticks

Personal Logo Instructions

Pull out the crayons, markers and construction paper (yes, real crayons and maybe some watercolors) and get busy!

1. To make your own logo, start with a blank sheet of paper.
2. Draw a circle and write your name in the center. You can write and draw inside and outside of your circle. Include "I am" statements like: I am peace, I am Love, I am the perfect expression of God.
3. Write your favorite mantras in and around your logo;; add anything that inspires you when you see it! If you don't have the words, draw something that represents who you are and who you are becoming.

For inspiration, try using these shapes in your design

Butterfly: rebirth, new life, transformation, new beginnings
Water: healing, deep emotions, infinite intelligence, abundance
Lion: courage, divine protection
Sun: energy, power
Spiral: creation, right path
Circle: wholeness, completion
Leaf: health, healing, life
Star: cosmic, enlightenment, peace
Heart: love, joy, oneness, connection
Fire: movement, action, spring
Earth: deeply rooted, comfortable within the self, fall
Air: thoughts, clarity, reflection, calm
Moon: rest, relaxation, intuition, divinity

Juice Recipe of the Day | Green Buddha

This juice is sweet enough with the pineapple, but I like ginger and apple together. If you are seeking more sugar-free options to sweeten your juice, consider adding low-glycemic fruit (green apples for example) or stevia. I use sweet leaf stevia (lemon drop). There are many varieties of stevia on the market. Check the ingredients. It shouldn't have more than stevia and water. If it does, they should be ingredients you understand and can pronounce.

Ingredients

1/4 inch ginger
1/4 lemon
1/4 pineapple
handful of spinach
1 cucumber
2 kale leaves and stems
optional: 1 apple

Instructions

1. Prep and peel your ingredients.
2. Juice fruit and vegetables in the order listed.

Day 14
Green Tea Goddess

If there was an award for best green juice taste, this one would win! It tastes like a juicy punch with fruits and veggies that love being together. You can tell!

There are lots of Green Goddess recipes. If you juice long enough (over a day) you'll make one up of your own!

Here's mine …

1/2 pineapple
big fistful of kale
big fistful of spinach
1 cucumber
1 orange
1 mango
1 nectarine

Instructions

1. Smile as you cleanse and prepare your ingredients.
2. Juice them while doing a happy dance.
3. Pour her in your chilled glass and sip.

At-Home Spa Treatments

Green Tea Body Butter

Ingredients

1/4 cup avocado butter (melted)
1 teaspoon chia seed oil
1/2 teaspoon shea nut oil
1/8 teaspoon calendula extract

1/8 teaspoon green tea extract
6 to 8 drops of bergamot, sandalwood, or palmarosa essential oil

Instructions

1. Add oils and extracts to melted butters.
2. Stir and allow to cool for up to 8 hours.
3. You may also chill this fruit and veggie butter in the refrigerator for about 2 hours.

Green Tea Sugar Scrub with Lemon

Ingredients

3 cups organic sugar
1 tablespoon fresh lemon juice
1 teaspoon lemon zest
1 teaspoon vitamin E oil
1 cup organic safflower oil
10 to 15 drops lemon essential oil
1 teaspoon lemon extract (fragrance)
1 teaspoon green tea extract

Instructions

Mix together sugar, lemon juice, zest, and vitamin E oil. Stir to gently blend the ingredients together.

Add the safflower oil slowly and stir. Add in the lemon extract and green tea extract. If you like your sugar scrubs to be drier, add less oil. I like mine to have slightly more oil than I think I need, so that it doesn't dry out as I use it. If this happens to your scrub, you may always add more oil and a tablespoon of honey for extra moisturizing power.

Add the lemon essential oil and lemon extract.

Day 15:
Give Yourself An Angel Card Reading

If you feel undeserving, it doesn't matter how much you study and practice manifestation methods. Until you feel deserving, you will sabotage your success and happiness.
—Doreen Virtue, Angels of Abundance: Heaven's 11 Messages to Help You Manifest Support, Supply, and Every Form of Abundance

I love angel cards, oracle cards, flower therapy decks, and fairy tarot to name a few. Angel Card Decks are great tools you can use to strengthen your mental, emotional, and spiritual awareness. It is an intuitive action that doesn't rely on your conscious mind. It's a way to receive messages from your soul. This includes your ancestors, angels, loved ones, dreams, feelings, sensations, insights, revelations, and even ancient memories—answers to enter into your current experience.

You Can Also Make Your Own…

Draw, paint, and create your own cards. Use whatever enters your mind: symbols, shapes, words, and capture them on paper. Use photos and pictures, anything that promotes the presence of peace.

Cut them out, shuffle, and pull. Create any number of cards from one to infinity! Any number of cards will work for this exercise.

Readings can be used to heal cognitive, behavioral, spiritual, and physiological imbalances that seem to have no other cause.

Other Benefits from Spiritual Readings:

- Strengthens your spiritual cognition, intuitive gifts, talents, and abilities.
- Opens and clears your connection to the Universal Source, Divine Intelligence, First Cause, Good Energy, Love, God, Allah, and any name you give this Eternal Power.
- A curative energy that heals you as you focus on it.

- Enhances your overall health and well-being.
- Opens you up to information you won't receive through any other channels.
- can be used as a cognitive, behavioral, and spiritual treatment

Give Yourself a Reading

One or more card decks (you can also download free card reading apps to get started; check the app store). There are butterfly, angel, tarot, gemstones, energy, warrior, goddess, you name it—there's a card deck for it!

Optional:

- **Candles** (represents the element of fire, burns away all that no longer serves us)
- **Incense** (represents the element of air, creates a sacred space, honors the inner self)
- **Bowl of water** (for clarity, clear thinking, and clear listening)
- **White sage** (clears negative energy, lifts spiritual vibration, provides spiritual protection)

Instructions

1. Select a card deck.
2. Center yourself with this breathing exercise:
   Gently blow out the air in your lungs. Breathe in through your nose and exhale through your mouth. Do this again: breathe in through your nose and exhale through your mouth. Focus on your exhale; empty all of the air out of your lungs by gently pulling your belly toward your back. This will cause you to take a nice, robust inhale.
3. Next, bring to mind a current situation or question you would like to have resolved. Be as specific as you can be, as your answer will match the question.

4. Now you are ready to begin the reading. Remove your deck from the box and turn your cards over so that you can see each image, angel, or affirmation.

5. Before shuffling, clear the energy of the deck by gently tapping it once with your left hand (the receiving hand).

6. Say hello to each card by greeting each one before shuffling. It's like saying, "Hello, angels? How are you today?"

7. Before selecting your three cards, call in your spiritual guides and archangels by saying:

   "I call forth my spiritual guides and advisors, guardian angels, and archangels. It is my intention to receive divine guidance through this reading with ease and effortlessness."

Mostly all card decks you purchase come with a guidebook that will give you greater details about each card and how to give yourself others readings. Always remember: you can't do it wrong!

The Three-Card Spread

1. Pull three cards
2. Keep cards facedown.
3. The card on the far left is where we begin. This card represents the immediate or distant past regarding the question or concern.
4. The card in the middle represents the current experience, what's going on now.
5. The card on the far right, the third card, represents the near future.
6. Read the messages on each card and study the images presented (colors, features, what thoughts and feelings are triggered as you look at the card).
7. Shuffle the deck.

You may notice a card pop up as if it's saying, "Pick me!" or you may simply choose to select the first three off the top; allow your intuition to lead you. The cards you select will be the right cards for you and the experience.

Juice Recipe of the Day | Soul Cleanse

Cucumbers are hydrating, excellent for healthy skin, hair, and nails, have warrior-level cancer-fighting properties (so do their friends carrots), and they're natural diuretics. For women, these beauty treatments help reduce inflammation both inside the body and out (place a few slices over your eyelids to soothe puffy eyes).

However...

It is the beautiful beetroot that has the extra womanly healing powers of this bountiful beverage! Beets are excellent for the heart and phenomenal for our reproductive organs. If you're into energy medicine, beetroot will balance and cleanse your sacral chakra on its own. *Try this:*

Soul Cleanse

1/2 beet
2 green apples
handful of broccoli
1 cucumber
handful of cilantro
1/2 lemon

Instructions

1. Add all of the ingredients to a high speed blender.
2. Blend for up to 1 minute or until smooth.
3. Pour into your favorite glass and enjoy!

Day 16
Wash Your Hair With Clay

Lavish Abundance

God is lavish, unfailing Abundance, the rich omnipresent substance of the universe. This All-providing Source of Infinite Prosperity is individualized as me—the reality of me.
—John Randolph Price, The Abundance Book

Define a few of the words in the following statement, so that it's in your language. Write it in a way you can see, feel, and experience—and like our natural products, go deep!

God is lavish, unfailing Abundance, the rich omnipresent substance of the universe. This All-providing Source of Infinite Prosperity is individualized as me—the reality of me.

I did a quick Google search and wrote some definitions to get you started.

- *Lavish* – sumptuously rich, elaborate, luxurious
- *Unfailing* – inexhaustible, endless, without error
- *Abundance* – fullness to overflowing, a great or plentiful amount
- *Rich* – plentiful, abundant, having a great deal of money or assets
- *Omnipresent* – present in all places at the same time
- *Universe* – the whole body of things and phenomena observed or postulated; the entire celestial cosmos
- *Infinite* – extending indefinitely; endless; immeasurably or inconceivably great or extensive: inexhaustible; subject to no limitation or external determination
- *Prosperity* – a successful, flourishing, or thriving condition; good fortune

But don't stop here. Define these words for yourself.

Once you have your definitions, rewrite this statement in *your* words based on *your* definitions.

Write it here:

_____

_____

_____

_____

_____

_____

_____

_____

Time to Apply

Think of the most difficult situation, event, or condition you are currently experiencing ...

Yes that one.

In your journal, write what's happening, what you're doing, and how it's making you feel.

Don't go over three minutes for this part of the exercise. Just give the highlights!

Then turn the page.

Write your new principle statement at the top and spend no more than five minutes writing about what you would like to see happen.

Think Abundantly

What do you really want to happen and what will it feel like when it happens?

Write in great detail how you will feel in the situation and what you're willing to let go of or do for this to happen. (For example, I'm willing to let go of the anger, I'm willing to forgive, I'm willing to let go of this relationship, I'm willing to ask for help …)

If you prefer, you may complete this activity in your video journal.

When you're finished, get up, put your favorite song on, and dance it out for a few minutes. If that's not an option, stretch, do some yoga, or have a hot love session (with yourself or your significant other).

Start now!

Juice Recipe of the Day | Abundance

This green juice is its own prosperity practice!

It's got kale, cucumber, spinach (my juice trifecta), pear, ginger, lemon and cabbage. An abundance of greens and nutrients that literally help you release old ideas, thoughts, feelings, memories, patterns, and conditions from your body.

You've probably heard of the health benefits of a juice with similar ingredients. What about how it makes you feel?

Here are the benefits you won't find anywhere else:

- promotes mental clarity and emotional balance
- increases awareness
- improves the ability to concentrate
- dissolves fear
- boosts energy and confidence
- helps release stress and feelings of overwhelm from your joints, muscles, and bones
- increases feelings of relaxation
- creates good energy in your body; clears the space so that you can receive more good

Taste Review

This juice is surprisingly sweet. There's just enough ginger for a teeny-weeny bit of spice but not so much that it overpowers the juice. For as many greens that are in this, you really can't tell by the taste.

Abundance

Ingredients

1/4 cabbage
3 kale leaves and stem
1 big handful of spinach
1/4 inch of ginger
1/4 lemon
1 pear

Instructions

1. Wash, prep, and peel your ingredients.
2. Juice and sip!

Remember:

If we want abundance, we must think abundantly. If we want wealth, we must believe we are wealthy. If we want to move beyond the struggle, hardships and restrictions we find in life, we must open our eyes and remember ... All that the Father has is mine!
—Iyanla Vanzant, *Acts of Faith*

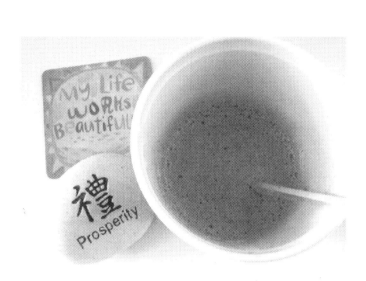

Meditate for 20 minutes.

Meditation is a state of being perfectly present in the moment. There is no past to dwell upon and no future to worry about. The relentless thoughts, fears, and concerns of the mind cease, giving way to deep peace and relaxation.

Meditation can produce feelings of tranquility, bliss, and clarity.

We always have access to this original state. This state of consciousness provides us with an abundance of benefits for body, mind, and soul.

The Benefits of Meditation

Meditation has countless potential benefits.

Physical benefits:

1. Relaxes the nervous system
2. Boosts the immune system
3. Increases oxygen and blood flow
4. Promotes better sleep
5. Reduces chronic pain
6. Reduces muscle tension
7. Reduces menstrual pain
8. Assists with weight loss
9. Reduces the risk of heart disease
10. Reduces dependence on medical care

Mental benefits:

1. Increased connectivity of the brain's right and left hemispheres
2. Better willpower
3. Reduces anxiety, worry, and stress
4. Reduces aggression

5. Improves focus
6. Increases problem-solving abilities
7. Increases creativity
8. Increases self-awareness and awareness in general
9. Helps to quit addictive behavior such as smoking or drugs
10. Allows you to better see the bigger picture

Spiritual benefits:

1. Improves intuition
2. Improves compassion
3. Creates a sense of inner peace, not dependent on external circumstance
4. Improves your relationship with yourself
5. Aligns body, mind, and soul
6. Helps us to forgive and let go of the past
7. Helps us to accept ourselves
8. Allows us to be here now in the present
9. Helps you to understand yourself and others
10. Allows us to experience a sense of oneness with existence/God/ the universe/Tao/Source

The #1 Goal of Meditation

While meditation is this state of presence and inner peace, there are countless methods used to reach it. These methods are meditation techniques, rather than the actual meditation itself. There are many meditation techniques, and it may take some experimentation until you find one that works for you.

Typically, the aim of meditation is to stay focused on a single thing in order to quiet the mind and open the space for inner silence. This may be physical sensations within the body, a mental visualization, or an object such as a candle or a single point in the distance of your vision like a tree or flower. The point of focus may be on nothing at all.

Crucially, the point of meditation is not to obtain or do anything; it is simply to stay in the present moment, which has become increasingly difficult for us amongst the many distractions of our modern world!

Key Features of Meditation
By Mo Gould, Reiki Therapist, Self-Esteem Coach

A common focal point of meditation is the breath. The practitioner sits and focuses on the sensation of the breath entering the body and leaving again. The rhythmic movements create a continuous distraction, allowing the mind to focus on stillness.

Some meditations use a mantra. Transcendental meditation (TM) relies on the practitioner repeating a specific word to create a single point of focus. This meditation is practiced for around twenty minutes, twice a day.

Some meditations require total stillness. There are meditations designed to push the limitations of discomfort, such as Vipassana in which its participants sit for ten hours a day, for ten consecutive days. This kind of practice allows the practitioner the opportunity to expand his or her physical and mental comfort zones.

Meditation is not limited to sitting. There is also standing meditation, a facet of Taoist Chi Gong, an ingenious exercise in which the practitioner stands still with arms outstretched, rooted to the earth like a tree. Unlike other forms of exercise, they actually accumulate energy rather than losing it. This may be more suited to people who wish to feel more physically present in their bodies during meditation practice.

Meditation is not limited to being still. The Sufis, the mystical branch of Islam, have whirling dervishes, where they practice spinning around continuously to enter the meditative state. There is also dynamic meditation, created by the mystic Osho with the intention of assisting modern people who sometimes struggle to sit still. In dynamic meditation, practitioners turn their focus to repeated and rhythmical movements. Chi gong and tai chi are other forms of moving meditation in which the focus is on the subtle movements of the physical body and the energy it creates.

Being mindful is meditation. Attention to any activity can be a form of meditation, such as washing up or doing other household chores. Mindfulness can be practiced at anytime, simply by being aware of one's thoughts and feelings. Meditation and mindfulness allow us to take a step back from the immediacy of our egoic minds and see them from a detached perspective, preventing us from getting lost in self-created problems and being able to better react to circumstance from a balanced position.

It can be fun to experiment with different meditation techniques. They are all designed to help us reach the same state of inner peace, and as there are so many, why settle on just one technique when you can experience a richness of variety?

A Brief Guide to Meditation for Beginners

Read these instructions two to three times to become familiar with them. You may even record them in your own voice. This way you don't have to stop during your practice.

1. Make sure you have the time and space to sit in silence. Turn off all distractions such as phones and social media.
2. Ideally set a timer with a pleasant notification sound for the practice. Shorter periods of time to meditate are easier for beginners to remain focused.
3. Sit in a comfortable position on a chair or on a cushion on the ground with your back straight.
4. Close your eyes and take a moment to scan your body, feeling for any sensations of tension. If you notice tension or discomfort, maneuver your body to make this comfortable.
5. Without forcing your breath, slow it down to a comfortable rhythm. Inhale through your nostrils and be aware of the sensation of your breath entering your nose.
6. Breathe deeply into your abdomen, feeling the expansion of your diaphragm as it fills with oxygen. During the inhalation, count slowly to ten.
7. Exhale gently out of your mouth and feel the oxygen rising up through your chest and leaving your body.
8. Maintain an even rhythm of inhalation and exhalation. Keep your focus on the movement of your breath.
9. Take note of the sensations you feel and listen to the stillness of the silence. Feel the steady pulsations and rhythms of your body.
10. Your mind will get distracted with thoughts. This is okay and to be expected. When this happens, simply return your awareness to your breath and the sensations in your body.

Remember this is about being, not doing. There is no such thing as a bad meditation practice. Don't worry when you get distracted; when you catch yourself, it increases your awareness. With practice, you will be able to maintain stillness for longer and longer periods and gradually uncover the tranquility, calm, and stillness that naturally exists within you.

Juice Recipe of the Day | Authentic Self

Wisdom, higher states of consciousness, and peace are a few effects of Authentic Self. Served over ice, you won't know whether you're drinking a fresh juicy punch or the natural wine from heaven!

Ingredients

1/2 pineapple
big fistful of kale
big fistful of spinach
1 cucumber
1 orange
1 mango
1 nectarine

Instructions:

1. Cleanse and prep your ingredients.
2. Juice them while doing a happy dance.

Day 18
Visualize It

Visualization, also referred to as guided imagery, is described as a mental process, use of imagination, or a variety of procedures used to change physiological, emotional, or behavioral responses.[39, 58] It is a practice that uses focused attention to visualize places, experiences, or objects that are perceived through all of the senses.

This noninvasive, safe technique[58] can be used to free your mind from distractions and competing thoughts.[89] Visualization has a proven effect on physiological processes that increase healthy immune function.[62]

This practice has also been found to:

- *facilitates calmness*[34]
- *increase creativity*
- *alleviate anxiety and pain*
- *improve quality of life*
- *reduce tension and relax the body*
- *encourages the receptivity of treatment*[47]

Today's Diet: Practice visualization.
Relaxation Activity: "See Thyself"

> *Move your body with a nice deep stretch. FInd a comfortable place to sit or lay, and turn on your favorite, soothing music.*

> *Close your eyes.*

> *See, feel, and imagine yourself 3 days from now. Fully immerse yourself in whatever comes to mind.*

> *Paint with a broad brush. See yourself having fulfilled everything you are cultivating right now.*

Use your sensory awareness to notice the seasons, the weather, the temperature of the places you are in. What does it feel like?

Be open to as many details as you can breathe in. What colors are you wearing? How is your hair??? What are you doing?

Play with this activity by visualizing yourself 3 months from now, 1 year from now, and 10 years from now.

When you are complete with this exercise, sit still and breathe for a few minutes.

Wiggle your fingers and toes. Give your body a nice stretch before you open your eyes.

Recipe of the Day | Emotional Detox: Passionate Patchouli

Relieve and prevent any feelings, thoughts, sensations, patterns, habits, or energies of depression with the deep, exotic, earthy scent of patchouli. Patchouli, a natural antidepressant that helps relieve insomnia and rejuvenates the skin. Today's recipe is wonderful for moving past any unconscious, conscious, and semiconscious hurts that may be hiding in your joints, bones and roots.

Massaging patchouli into your scalp and skin:

- helps transmute all forms of mental pain
- stimulates creativity
- improves concentration
- repels stress
- increases hair growth and fullness
- Improves the quality of your sleep
- clears all repressed, suppressed, and unexpressed fear

Patchouli's secret -- it works as a natural cell rejuvenator in the body, and is often used to treat acne, eczema, dandruff, cracked skin, and athlete's foot.

Passionate Patchouli Scalp and Skin Rejuvenator with Chia Seed and Apricot Oil

Ingredients

2 drops rose essential oil
2 drops bergamot essential oil
4 drops patchouli essential oil
2 drops sandalwood essential oil
1/4 cup apricot kernel oil
1/4 cup passion fruit oil
1 teaspoon watermelon seed oil
1 teaspoon chia seed oil
1 teaspoon vitamin e oil
4-ounce bottle

Instructions

Add all of the ingredients to the bottle and gently wiggle to mix. Oh, and you can gently shake the bottle too! This is harmonizing energy balancing blend is also perfect for use as an after bath oil.

Day 19
Master the Relaxation Response

The relaxation response (RR) is an effective self-help technique that has improved and/or eliminated conditions such as anxiety, morning sickness, cardiac arrhythmias, and severe forms of pain.[6]

While researching advanced forms of meditation, a cardiologist by the name of Herbert Benson, MD (2000) started observing Tibetan monks and practitioners of transcendental meditation (TM) for his research. He was seeking options other than invasive treatments for his patients. through his years of practice, He argued that self-care was as important to healing as the other medical treatments and prescriptions in medical care. Benson (2000) found that TM practitioners experienced a profound state of rest that was associated with physiological changes:

> "Such as decreased oxygen consumption, heart rate, respiratory rate, arterial blood lactate, and increased frequency and intensity of electroencephalographic alpha and theta waves, with decreased sympathetic nervous system activity" (p. 312).[8]

These physiological changes led to a relaxed state that also increased blood flow to the brain and the skin. This created feelings of warmth and "rested mental alertness" (Borysenko, 1987). Benson (2000) called this relaxed state the relaxation response.

Benson (2000) discovered that any form of mental concentration practiced for ten to twenty minutes could elicit this "innate, hypothalamic mechanism" that could improve mental and medical conditions.[6, 8]

He created a four-step process based on his research, observations, and study of major religions (that utilized relaxation techniques similar to TM) that could elicit the relaxation response. This is important for us today because we're going to practice activating this response on our own. You can access this response at any time. To practice this technique, follow these steps:

1. *The first step is to focus on one's breathing and anchor the mind with a word, phrase, or sound.*
2. *The second step is to have a "passive, nonjudgmental attitude" (p. 312)[7] so that the person does not become distracted by the daily cares or concerns of the mind.*
3. *The third step is to get into a comfortable position, close the eyes, and relax the muscles from head to toe (also known as the body scan).*
4. *The final step is to make sure to be in a quiet environment (p. 312).[7] [8]*

Smoothie Recipe of the Day | Moody Blues

An all-natural smoothie packed with vitamins, mood-balancing phytonutrients, and an abundance of antioxidants, this drink can do everything from reducing feelings of depression to boosting your energy levels.

Ingredients

1 cup fresh or frozen blueberries
1 handful raspberries
1 ripe banana, sliced
1 cup crushed ice
1/2 cup coconut water (or your favorite seed or nut milk)
1 teaspoon maca root powder
optional: 1 teaspoon your favorite sweetener

Instructions

1. Add the blueberries, raspberries, banana, maca root powder, crushed ice, and coconut water to your blender.

2. Blend ingredients for about 1 minute or until smooth. If you like your smoothie thicker, add less water.

3. Pour into a special glass, a wine glass even, and make it uniquely special. Enjoy each sip. Think about all of the good things you're doing for your mind and body.

As you enjoy this drink, repeat the following affirmation silently or out loud in front of a mirror:

"I love and approve of myself just as I am."

Relaxation Activity | Make Hair Butter

Organic Hair Butter

1 tablespoon organic shea butter
1/2 tablespoon organic coconut oil
1/2 tablespoon organic olive oil

Instructions

1. Simply melt the ingredients down in a heat-safe container or in a small pot on the lowest heat setting.
2. Remove from heat and let cool for 10 minutes.
3. Pour into a sealable jar.
4. Place in your refrigerator for up to 20 minutes, or in your freezer for 10 minutes.

Additional Options:

Add any (or all) of these options for a light, all-natural butter:

- 2 to 4 drops palmarosa essential oil
- 1 teaspoon aloe vera gel
- 1/2 tablespoon organic cocoa butter

Notes

This organic hair butter recipe won't weigh your hair down, provides your curls with deep moisture, eliminates frizz, and can be ready to use within a few minutes.

My kind of hair butter!

This recipe makes about 2 ounces. If you need more, it's super simple to double. It's also a great moisturizer for hands, feet, and twinkly toes.

Your butter will be firm but soft to the touch. It should easily melt on your fingers and into your hair.

Day 20
Grow Your Hair With Carrots

Hello, Magnificence!

Today's recipe is all about calming your system from the inside out. Raw carrot juice energizes your joints, enlivens the organs and tissues, purifies the blood, and boosts your immune system against all forms of infection. It's also excellent for the prevention of spiritual autism: the inability to speak your truth, balance your emotions, and accept your divinity. They're also good for your spiritual vision, your intuition, and ability to hear, see, know, and easily interpret divine guidance.

Most of us have heard about the goodness of carrots in strengthening and improving vision. Carrot seed oil is a purifying oil that has been used to treat skin irritations, as a natural emollient, and as a treatment for acne. It's also phenomenal for hair growth.

Did you know that carrots are also phenomenal for your heart?

They lower your risk of heart disease and are a huge anticancer advocate in your body.

Take a curative approach to health today and go crazy with carrots!

I Heart Carrots!

After your morning meditation, make this delicious orange juice abundantly alive with carrots.

Carrots are a root vegetable packed with beta-carotene, fiber, and vitamins A, B1, B2, B3, B6, biotin, and vitamin K. They're known for being orange but may also be white, purple, yellow, and red.

Benefits of this crunchy delight include:

- helps reduce your risk of heart attack
- lowers blood pressure
- helps repair and rejuvenate skin tissue (making it a powerful antiaging veggie)
- improves eyesight
- strengthens hair
- reduces your risk of stroke
- stimulates hair growth
- helps regulate blood sugar levels
- boosts your immune system

"I Heart Carrots" Juice Recipe

4 big, happy carrots
1 big, beautiful orange
4 kale leaves
1/2 mango
1/4 fresh pineapple

Wash and prep your ingredients.
Juice them with a smile!

This juice tastes just like orange pineapple juice. If you have little ones, they won't be able to tell there's kale hanging out in there!
Chill a glass for 15 minutes in the freezer, pour, and enjoy!

Bonus Recipe | Frozen "I Heart Carrots"

Have this juice for dessert! Add juice to your favorite ice-cream maker. You can even pour it into a sandwich bag. Put it in the freezer, and it's ready in about four hours.

Before Evening Meditation . . .

If you have some extra carrots and olive oil, make a rich batch of carrot oil. Carrot oil is an antiviral, antiseptic, antioxidant oil that moisturizes hair and skin, relieves stress, stimulates hair growth, and soothes muscle pain.

Homemade carrot oil is way better than anything you'll ever buy in the store, and if you have vanilla essential oil around, it will smell like carrot cake! If you don't have vanilla, you can always use your favorite essential oil for fragrance.

Carrot Cake Carrot Oil Recipe

You Will Need:

grater
crockpot
strainer
16-ounce bottle or mason jar
*may also be simmered on the stove in a small pot on the lowest heat setting

Ingredients

3 carrots
1 cup of olive oil
1 cup coconut oil
4 to 6 drops vanilla essential oil or 1/2 vanilla bean

Instructions

1. Wash and prepare your carrots.
2. Grate and add them to your crockpot.

3. Add your oil(s).
4. Put your crockpot on the warm setting. Let it simmer for up to 2 hours. If your crockpot gets too hot, simmer on warm for 30 minutes.
5. Strain the carrots and goodies from the oil.
6. Pour into a squeeze bottle with top.
7. Use lavishly for natural hair styling, as a skin moisturizer, and as after-exercise massage oil (for tired muscles).

Day 21
Measure Your Results...With Hummus!

Congratulations! You've completed the Twenty-One-Day Relaxation Diet!

Take the same assessments that you completed at the beginning of the diet. Compare your results. This will give you a visible means of seeing the effects of the relaxation diet.

After the Diet

1. Complete the Perceived Stress Scale and the Authentic Happiness Inventory.
2. If you took a starting weight at the beginning, weigh yourself today and write down your results.
3. Snap a photo for your "after" results.
4. Let me see you! Post your photo to LavishlyNatural.com/goddess
5. Keep going! Now that the diet is over, don't stop! Daily relaxation in all forms has a preventive and curative effect on your health.

Post-Diet Assessments

- **The Perceived Stress Scale (PSS)**
  http://www.psy.cmu.edu/~scohen/PSS.html

  For more about the PSS, visit Dr. Sheldon Cohen at Carnegie Mellon University:
  http://www.psy.cmu.edu/~scohen/

- **Authentic Happiness Inventory,** University of Pennsylvania
  https://www.authentichappiness.sas.upenn.edu

Heavenly Hummus Recipe for Good Hair Days

I didn't want this diet to end without sharing the best hummus recipe on the planet. Made with chickpeas, garlic, and lemon (the divine trio), it's good for you and tastes great with chips and on a sandwich!

This recipe comes is from a blog post when I was still finding delicious recipes my son could eat—that were also easy to make. When DJ was placed on a gluten-free, plant-based, nut-free, and sugar-free diet, there weren't very many foods he liked to eat. This recipe saved the day for a quick family snack that's nice to the gut and great for your hair!

Blog Post from EricaKKing.com, April 20, 2014

So, my son and I have been on a blue corn chips thing.

He loves them, they're on the Body Ecology Diet, and they're good.

The problem is, every time I eat them, I have a craving for hummus.

At our old home, we lived across the street from a Fresh and Easy, and they made the best hummus.

I knew I could make it myself, but after searching for tahini, for longer than I care to share, I finally found some sesame seeds and got to it! I had no idea tahini was sesame seed paste.

We eat lots of legumes in our home, so chickpeas (garbanzo beans) are always in my cabinet.

Garbanzo beans:

- are high in fiber
- help regulate fat regulation (which lowers LDL cholesterol and total cholesterol)
- helps balance emotions

- are filled with insoluble fiber (which is good for your digestive tract and colon)
- keep you full and decrease your appetite (specifically for processed foods)
- relieves stress and inner anxiety
- are filled with a whopping 273% of molybdenum

What Is Molybdenum?

The American Cancer Society (2016) describes this essential element as necessary for "biological processes, possibly including development of the nervous system, waste processing in the kidneys, and energy production in cells."

Pretty powerful element—right?

Chickpeas are also high in:

- manganese (84.5 percent)
- folate (70.5 percent)
- copper (64.4 percent)

Manganese is a trace mineral that helps with bone production, skin health, blood sugar balance, and protection against free radical damage (which can cause asthma and skin problems).

Enjoy this delicious healthy dip for your favorite chip!

Heavenly Hummus Recipe

Ingredients

1 (15-ounce) can chickpeas (garbanzo beans) with liquid
2 tablespoons raw sesame seeds

1 tablespoon olive oil
2 tablespoons lemon juice
1 garlic clove
1/2 teaspoon cumin
1 teaspoon tamari sauce (or soy sauce)
*optional: salt to taste

Instructions

1. Add ingredients to your blender in the order listed.
2. Blend on high for 1 to 2 minutes or until smooth and creamy.
3. Transfer to a sealable container or straight to your dip bowl.

Notes

I like to add a little more olive oil, maybe two tablespoons (total) for extra creamy awesomeness! For more, view the online version of this recipe at EricaKKing.com/heavenlyhummus

Juice of the Day | Sweet Mango Carrot Smoothie

Ingredients

1 whole banana
2 large carrots
1/2 sweet potato
1 mango
1/4 lemon
optional: fresh wheatgrass

Instructions

1. Wash and prep your fruit and veggies.
2. Juice or blend your ingredients.

Relaxation Activity: Coach Yourself (Self-Coaching Exercise)

Begin with a centering exercise.
Close your eyes.
Inhale through your mouth; exhale through your mouth.
Slowly inhale, taking in as much air as you can
and exhale with a cool ahhhhhhh.
Do this again: slowly inhale taking in as much air as
you can, and then taking in more, even a few extra sips,
and exhale with an even cooler ahhhhhhhhh.
Allow your breathing to return to its normal rhythm.
Using a notebook or journal, pick up your pen and write with your
non-dominant hand (the hand you usually don't write with).
Set a goal for your session and begin.
Write the first question that comes to mind. Write
this question with your dominant hand.
Listen for the answer. You do not have to make one up.
Write the answer with your non-dominant hand.
Continue your Q&A until there are no questions left for you to answer.

Congratulations!

You have completed the Twenty-One-Day Relaxation Diet! You have reset, recalibrated, renewed, recommitted to, and resumed every good thing in abundance—health, wealth, peace, joy, and great hair! The healing has been thorough and complete, swift and just. For the next few days and weeks, be aware that healing will still be taking place. Keep writing about your daily practice. Continue to relax or meditate for at least ten minutes a day.

Consistency is the cure!

You are healthy not because I say so but because you can measure your own health outcomes with ease, accuracy, and grace.

I join with the World Health Organization,* who defines health as

"a state of complete physical, mental and social well-being and not merely the absence of disease or infirmity."[69]

Repeat this spiritual treatment with me, out loud and looking into your own eyes:

"I am in a complete state of physical, mental, social, spiritual, cosmic, cellular, energetic well-being. I am perfect health, made in the image and likeness, thoughts and idea of God. I speak health and claim this divine energy in and as all I am."

So be it.

And so it is.

*"Preamble to the Constitution of the World Health Organization as adopted by the International Health Conference, New York, 19–22 June, 1946; signed on 22 July 1946 by the representatives of 61 States (Official Records of the World Health Organization, no. 2, p. 100) and entered into force on 7 April 1948. The Definition has not been amended since 1948."

Appendix A

The Lavishly Natural Shopping List

It's time to assess what you already have in your healing spa and go shopping! Here's a grocery list of the ingredients, butters, and oils used in this book. You don't need to buy everything on this list to get started. Most of the items can be found in your local markets and grocery stores. I've also included my favorite places to shop for these ingredients at the end of the list.

Butters

avocado butter
cocoa butter
cupuacu butter
kokum butter
illipe butter
mango butter
shea butter

Clays

bentonite clay
rhassoul clay

Essential Oils

atlas cedar wood essential oil
basil essential oil
grapefruit essential oil
rosemary essential oil
lavender essential oil
lemon essential oil
orange essential oil
palmarosa essential oil
peppermint essential oil
sandalwood essential oil
rose essential oil
rosehip seed essential oil
rosewood essential oil
vanilla essential oil
ylang ylang essential oil

Botanicals and Extracts

aloe vera extract
amla powder
calendula extract
calendula flowers
catnip leaves
chamomile leaves and flowers
comfrey root
dandelion root
dried red or pink roses
dried rosemary
fenugreek powder
fenugreek seeds
hibiscus flowers
hibiscus powder
horsetail powder
lavender flowers

linden leaf powder

marshmallow root powder

soap nuts

whole vanilla beans (or vanilla powder)

Food-Based Ingredients

aloe vera gel

aloe vera juice

apple pie spice

bananas

brown rice

cactus leaves

chia seeds

coconut cream

coconut oil

coconut milk

coconut water

distilled water

flaxseeds

hemp seeds

fresh or dried mint

raw apple cider vinegar

raw honey

spirulina

Oils

apricot kernel oil

avocado oil

castor oil

chia seed oil

hemp seed oil

rice bran oil

shea nut oil

rice bran oil

olive oil
passion fruit oil
peach kernel oil
pumpkin seed oil
safflower oil
sunflower oil
vitamin E

Beeswax Substitutes

candelilla wax
caranuba wax
rice bran wax
sunflower wax

Optional Extras

raw agave syrup
aloe vera leaves
coconut manna
matcha green tea
molasses
optiphen (preservative)
vegetable glycerin
xanthan gum

Where to Buy

There are a gazillion sites that sell awesome organic ingredients. Here are a few of my favorites:

Amazon.com

If I can't find it locally, I turn to the big A for almost everything else. Hair clips, plastic bags (for deep conditioning), and NOW's Shea Nut Oil are a few go-to items I like to order from here.

Brambleberry.com

They have the absolute best fragrance oils for your recipes, and this is the place for your chia seed oil, green tea extract, and calendula extract. They offer a range of sizes to choose from, and if you're into soap making or making your own all-mineral makeup, this is the place! They offer high-quality butters, oils, and essential oils. They also like to include free samples each month in your order. Plus, their Grapefruit Bellini fragrance will change your life.

Butters-N-Bars.com

They have the best shea butter on the planet—hands down! It's soft and luscious and mixes extremely well in your homemade formulations. Butters-N-Bars offers carrier oils, essential oils, henna, fragrance oils, and packing/storage containers. Their containers are sturdy and last forever!

Encha.com

Not all *matcha green teas* are the same. There are a few things to look for before investing in this tea meditation:

color, grade, and affordability. Your green tea should be bright green in color. You'll want an organic, ceremonial grade (the first cut of the tea leaves; more powerful than other grades). You shouldn't have to spend an arm and a headful of hair to have it! I've bought my tea from a few places, but I always come back to Encha. They have 3 different ceremonial grades, great recipes *(their encha pancakes are delicious),* and affordable tea *(with really cool tea accessories).* Their ceremonial grade mixes well with coconut milk AND water.

Hennasooq.com

Henna Sooq not only specializes in the best body-art-quality henna, they also offer handmade soap, a hair gloss that will give life to tired, dry curls, and my personal favorite, red raj henna. If you are a henna head like I used to be, this will become your only source for all things henna!

MountainRoseHerbs.com

Specializes in organic herbs, flowers, spices, extracts, teas, hydrosols, tinctures, scales, and everything you need to make your own lip butters and healing recipes. Affordable pricing and high-quality ingredients.

Organic-Creations.com

Looking for an alternative to beeswax (their candelilla wax is a 1:1 substitute that's awesome), they'll have it! They specialize in raw ingredients, carrier oils, butters, body-care ingredients, cosmetics, essential oils, and crystals.

Teliaoils.com

Telia Oils offers those oils you can't seem to find anywhere else. I discovered them on Etsy when I couldn't find broccoli seed oil anywhere else. They have so many unique and luscious oils to choose from, I could live there. I love their watermelon, oregano, and of course broccoli seed oils.

TheSage.com

I started shopping at The Sage when Martha Stewart said she bought her dried lavender flowers from them. I've been hooked ever since! They have everything, and I mean everything, you need to make, store, and even sell your own natural creations. In addition to almost every carrier oil, essential, dried herb and extract, they also sell bottles, containers, jars, molds, lip butter tubes, and more. I love infusing my oils with their flowers because they're so fragrant.

INDEX

REFERENCES

1   Akihisa, T., Kojima, N., Kikuchi, T., Yasukawa, K. Tokuda, H., Masters, E., Manosroi, A., and Manosroi, J., "Anti-inflammatory and chemopreventive effects of triterpene cinnamates and acetates from shea fat," *Journal of Oleo Science* 59, no. 6 (2010): 273–80.

2   Akihisa, T., Kojima, N., Katoh, N., Kikuchi, T., Fukatsu, M. Shimizu, N., and Masters, E. T., "Triacylglycerol and triterpene ester composition of shea nuts from seven African countries," *Journal of Oleo Science* 60, no. 8 (2011): 385–391.

3   Albright, M. B., "Organic Foods Are Tastier and Healthier, Study Finds," (2014, July 14), retrieved from http://theplate.nationalgeographic.com/2014/07/14/organic-foods-are-tastier-and-healthier-study-finds/.

4   Barrett, R. K. and Barrett, J. A., "Facts: Dandelion Tea Benefits," (2009), retrieved from DandelionTea.org.

5   Bell, P., Walshe, I. H., Davison, G. W., Stevenson, E. J., Howatson, G., "Recovery facilitation with Montmorency cherries following high-intensity, metabolically challenging exercise," *Applied Physiology, Nutrition and Metabolism* 40, no. 4 (2015): 414–423.

6   Benson, H., *The Relaxation Response* (New York: HarperCollins Publishers Inc./ Quill, 2000).

7   Bonadonna, R., "Meditation's impact on chronic illness," *Holistic Nursing Practice* 17, no. 6 (2003): 309–319.

8   Borysenko, J., *Minding the Body, Mending the Mind* (New York, NY: Bantam Books, 1987).

9   Brannon, L. and Feist, J., *Health Psychology: An Introduction To Behavior and Health* (Belmont, CA: Wadsworth/Thompson, 2004).

10 Brogan, K., "Two Foods That May Sabotage Your Brain," (2015), retrieved from http://kellybroganmd.com/two-foods-may-sabotage-brain/.

11 Bullo M, Lamuela-Raventos R and Salas-Salvado J., "Mediterranean Diet and Oxidation: Nuts and Olive Oil as Important Sources of Fat and Antioxidants. Current Topics in 15," *Medicinal Chemistry* 11, no. 14 (2011): 1797–1810, http://

benthamscience.com/journals/current-topics-in-medicinal-chemistry/
volume/11/issue/14/page/1797/.

12 "Calendula | Uses, Side Effects, Interactions and Warnings," WebMD, retrieved
from http://www.webmd.com/vitamins-supplements/ingredientmono-235-
calendula.aspx?activeingredientid=235andactiveingredientname=
calendulaandprint=true.

13 Sources of Gluten. (n.d.). Celiac Disease Foundation. Retrieved from https://
celiac.org/live-gluten-free/glutenfreediet/sources-of-gluten/

14 Centini, M., Tredici, M. R., Biondi, N., Buonocore, A., Maffei Facino, R., and
Anselmi, C., "Thermal mud maturation: organic matter and biological activity,"
International Journal of Cosmetic Science 37, no. 3 (2015): 339–347, doi:10.1111/
ics.12204.

15 Chaudhary, K., "Herb of the Month: Dandelion," (2013, April 9), retrieved from
http://blog.doctoroz.com/oz-experts/herb-of-the-month-dandelion.

16 Clare, B. A., Conroy, R. S., and Spelman, K., "The Diuretic Effect in Human
Subjects of an Extract of Taraxacum officinale Folium over a Single Day,"
Journal of Alternative and Complementary Medicine 15, no. 8 (2009): 929–934, http://
doi.org/10.1089/acm.2008.0152.

17 "Dandelion: Uses and Side Effects," WebMD, retrieved from http://www.
webmd.com/vitamins-supplements/ingredientmono-706-dandelion.
aspx?activeingredientid=706and.

18 Drobot, J. and Thom, D., "Castor oil: An essential for health," Marion Institute,
retrieved from http://www.marioninstitute.org/biological-medicine-network/
resources/articles/castor-oil-essential-health.

19 Deckro, G. R., Ballinger, K. M., Hoyt, M., Wilcher, M., Dusek, J., Myers,
P., Greenberg, B., Rosenthal, D. S., and Benson, H., "The evaluation of a
mind/body intervention to reduce psychological distress and perceived stress
in college students," *Journal of American College Health* 50, no. 6 (2002): 281–287.

20 Ethylparaben. (2017). Retrieved from https://www.ewg.org/skindeep/
ingredient/702355/ETHYLPARABEN/#

21 Evangelista, M. P., Abad-Casintahan, F., and Lopez-Villafuerte, L., "The effect
of topical virgin coconut oil on SCORAD index, transepidermal water loss, and
skin capacitance in mild to moderate pediatric atopic dermatitis: a randomized,
double-blind, clinical trial," *International Journal of Dermatology* 53, no. 1 (2014):
100–108. doi:10.1111/ijd.12339.

22 EWG (2016). Butylparaben. Retrieved from http://www.ewg.org/skindeep/
ingredient/700868/BUTYLPARABEN/.

23 EWG (2016). Dimethicone. Retrieved from http://www.ewg.org/skindeep/
ingredient/702011/DIMETHICONE/.

24 EWG (2016). Ethylparaben. Retrieved from http://www.ewg.org/skindeep/
ingredient/702355/ETHYLPARABEN/.

25 EWG (2016). Methylparaben. Retrieved from http://www.ewg.org/skindeep/ingredient/703937/METHYLPARABEN/.

26 EWG (2016). Propylparaben. Retrieved from http://www.ewg.org/skindeep/ingredient/705335/PROPYLPARABEN/.

27 FDA (2016). Parabens in Cosmetics. Retrieved from http://www.fda.gov/cosmetics/productsingredients/ingredients/ucm128042.htm.

28 Fillmore, C., *The Revealing Word, A Dictionary of Metaphysical Terms* (Unity Village, MI: Unity Books, 1997).

29 Firpo-Cappiello, R., "16 Simple Healing Foods," (2014, May 22), retrieved from http://www.prevention.com/food/food-remedies/16-simple-healing-foods-0/slide/2.

30 Gates, D. and Schatz, L., *The Body Ecology Diet. Discovering Your Health and Rebuilding Your Immunity* (Carlsbad, CA: Hay House, Inc., 2011).

31 Gladstar, R., *Family Herbal: A Guide to Living Life with Energy, Vitality, and Health* (North Adams, MA: Storey Books, 2001).

32 Grieser, G., "Spice of the Month: Vanilla," (2012), retrieved from http://www.rethinkingcancer.org/blog/spice-of-the-month-vanilla/.

33 Grover, H. S., Deswal, H., Singh, Y., and Bhardwaj, A., "Therapeutic effects of amla in medicine and dentistry: A review," *Journal of Oral Research and Review* 7, no. 2 (2015): 65–68, doi:10.4103/2249-4987.172498.

34 Gruzelier, J., Levy, J., Williams, J., and Henderson, D., "Self-hypnosis and exam stress: comparing immune and relaxation-related imagery for influences on immunity, health and mood," *Contemporary Hypnosis* 18, no. 2 (2001): 73–86.

35 Gunners, K., "Why Modern Wheat Is Worse Than Older Wheat," (2016), retrieved from https://authoritynutrition.com/modern-wheat-health-nightmare/.

36 Hook I, McGee A, and Henman, M., "Evaluation of dandelion for diuretic activity and variation in potassium content," *International Journal of Pharmacognosy* 31, no. 1 (1993): 29–34.

37 Inner Visions Institute of Spiritual Development, (2001), Meditation Practices and Principles MPP/01, Life Experiences and the Impact of Chakra Energy within the Body, class handout, Silver Spring, MD.

38 Israel. M. O., "Effects of Topical and Dietary Use of Shea Butter on Animals," *American Journal of Life Sciences* 2, no. 5 (2014): 303–307, doi: 10.11648/j.ajls.20140205.18.

39 Joseph, A., "The impact of imagery on cognition and belief systems," *European Journal of Clinical Hypnosis* 5, no. 4 (2004): 12–15.

40 Keville, K., "Aromatherapy: Cedarwood," (2007, April 30), retrieved from http://health.howstuffworks.com/wellness/natural-medicine/aromatherapy/aromatherapy-cedarwood.htm.

41 Keville, K. and Green, M., *Aromatherapy: A Complete Guide to the Healing Art*, 2nd edition (New York: Crossing Press, 2008).

42 King, E. W., "The Effectiveness of an Internet-based Stress Management Program in the Prevention of Postpartum Stress, Anxiety, and Depression for New Mothers," Doctoral dissertation (2009), retrieved from ProQuest Dissertations and Theses, (UMI No. 3355047).

43 Lawless, J., "Cedarwood," *The Illustrated Encyclopedia of Essential Oils* (Rockport, MA: Element Books, 1995).

44 "Lavender: Uses, Side Effects, Interactions and Warnings," WebMD, retrieved from http://www.webmd.com/vitamins-supplements/ingredientmono-838-lavender.aspx?activeingredientid=838.

45 Manning, J., "Apple Cider Vinegar and Your Health," (2011, October 4), retrieved from http://www.webmd.com/diet/obesity/features/apple-cider-vinegar-and-health?page=2#2.

46 Maxwell, R. W. (2009). The physiological foundation of yoga chkra expression. Journal of Religion & Science, 44(4), 807-824.

47 McCaffrey, R. and Taylor, N., "Effective anxiety treatment prior to diagnostic cardiac catheterization," *Holistic Nursing Practice* 19, no. 2 (2005): 70–73.

48 McGarey, W. A., *The Oil That Heals: A Physician's Successes with Castor Oil Treatments* (Virginia Beach, VA: A.R.E. Press, 2004).

49 McKierman, J., "Hemp Seed Oil: The New Healthy Oil," (2012, June 1), retrieved from http://www.naturalnews.com/036039_hemp_seeds_oil_EFAs.html.

50 Mercola, J., "Vanilla Oil: The sweet smell of nature," (2016), retrieved from http://articles.mercola.com/herbal-oils/vanilla-oil.aspx.

51 Mercola, J., "What the Research Really Says about Apple Cider Vinegar," (2009, June 2), retrieved from http://articles.mercola.com/sites/articles/archive/2009/06/02/apple-cider-vinegar-hype.aspx.

52 Meyerowitz, S., *Wheatgrass: The Complete Guide to Using Grasses to Revitalize Your Health* (Great Barrington, MA: Sproutman Publications, 2006).

53 Michalum, N. and Michalum, M. V., *Milady's Skin Care and Cosmetic Ingredients Dictionary*, 3rd edition (Clifton Park, NY: Milady/Cengage Learning, 2010).

54 Naveed. A., Shahiq, U. Z., Barat, A. K., Muhammad, N. A., and Muhammad, A. E., "Calendula Extract: Effects on mechanical parameters of human skin," *Acta Poloniae Pharmaceutica—Drug Research* 68, no. 5 (2011): 693–701, [Abstract] http://www.ncbi.nlm.nih.gov/pubmed/21928714.

55 Pruimboom, L. and de Punder, K., "The opioid effects of gluten exorphins: asymptomatic celiac disease. Journal of Health," Population and Nutrition 33, no. 24 (2015), DOI: 10.1186/s41043-015-0032-y.

56 Rele, A. S. and Mohile, R. B., "Effects of mineral oil, sunflower oil, and coconut oil on prevention of hair damage," *Journal of Cosmetic Science* 54 (2003): 175–192.

57 Riley, Tess, "Spirulina; A luxury healthfood and panacea for malnutrition," (2014, September 12), Retrieved from http://www.theguardian.com/sustainable-business/2014/sep/12/spirulina-health-food-panacea-malnutrition.

58 Roffe, L., Schmidt, K., and Ernst, E., "A systematic review of guided imagery as an adjuvant cancer therapy," *Psycho-Oncology* 14 (2005): 607–617.

59 Schiller, C. and Schiller, D., *The Aromatherapy Encyclopedia: A Concise Guide To Over 385 Plant Oils* (Laguna Beach, CA: Basic Health Publications, Inc., 2008). Stefanato, C. M., "Histopathology of alopecia: a clinicopathological approach to diagnosis," *Histopathology* 56, no. 1 (2010): 24–38, doi:10.1111/j.1365-2559.2009.03439.x.

60 Taghipour, K., Tatnall, F., and Orton, D., "Allergic axillary dermatitis due to hydrogenated castor oil in a deodorant," *Contact Dermatitis* (01051873) 58, no. 3 (2008): 168–169, doi:10.1111/j.1600-0536.2007.01160.x.

61 Tsao, A. S., Kim, E. S., and Hong, W. K., "Chemoprevention of cancer," *CA: A Cancer Journal for Clinicians* 54, no. 3 (2004): 1542–4863.

62 Utay, J. and Miller, M., "Guided imagery as an effective therapeutic technique: brief review of its history and efficacy research," *Journal of Instructional Psychology* 33, no. 1 (2006): 40–43.

63 Virtue, D., *Butterfly Oracle Cards for Life Changes* (Carlsbad, CA: Hay House, Inc., 2016).

64 Virtue. D., *Divine Guidance, How to Have a Dialogue with God and Your Guardian Angels* (Los Angeles, CA: Renaissance Books, 1998).

65 Virtue. D. and Reeves, R., *Flower Therapy Oracle Cards*. Carlsbad (CA: Hay House, Inc., 2013).

66 Wani, S.A., Kumar, P., "Fenugreek: A review on its nutraceutical properties and utilization in various food products," *Journal of the Saudi Society of Agricultural Sciences* (2016), http://dx.doi.org/10.1016/j.jssas.2016.01.007.

67 WHFoods.com, "Olive Oil, Extra Virgin," (2016), retrieved from http://www.whfoods.com/genpage.php?tname=foodspiceanddbid=132.

68 Williams, L. B., and Haydel, S. E., "Evaluation of the medicinal use of clay minerals as antibacterial agents," *International Geology Review* 52, no. 7/8 (2010): 745–770, http://doi.org/10.1080/00206811003679737.

69 World Health Organization, "Preamble to the Constitution of the World Health Organization as adopted by the International Health Conference, New York, 19–22 June, 1946; signed on 22 July 1946 by the representatives of 61 States (Official Records of the World Health Organization, no. 2, p. 100) and entered into force on 7 April 1948," (2003), retrieved from http://www.who.int/about/definition/en/print.html.

70 Yang, C., and Cotsarelis, G., "Review of hair follicle dermal cells," *Journal of Dermatological Science* 57, no. 1 (2010): 2, http://doi.org/10.1016/j.jdermsci.2009.11.005.

71   Zague, V., Polacow, M. O., Pires-de-Campos, M. M., and Leonardi, G. R., "Evaluation of the ultrasound influence in the cutaneous penetration of d-panthenol: testin vitro," *Journal of Cosmetic Dermatology* 4, no. 1 (2005): 29–33, doi:10.1111/j.1473-2165.2005.00156.x.

72   Zarai, Z., Ben Chobba, I., Ben Mansour, R., Békir, A., Gharsallah, N., and Kadri, A., "Essential oil of the leaves of Ricinus communis L.: In vitro cytotoxicity and antimicrobial properties," *Lipids in Health and Disease* 11, no. 1 (2012): 102–108, doi:10.1186/1476-511X-11-102.

73   Zelman, K. M. (2016). The Truth About Kale. WebMD. Retrieved from http://www.webmd.com/food-recipes/kale-nutrition-and-cooking#1

ABOUT THE AUTHOR

Erica K. King, PhD, is a health psychologist and certified angel card reader. Her work in stress management has helped women and men heal from depression, anxiety, stress, addiction, and hair loss. Erica holds Bachelor of Arts Degree in Communications from Western Kentucky University, a Master of Arts Degree in Counseling from Hampton University, and a Doctorate in Health Psychology from Walden University. She is a Member of the American Psychological Association, the Society for the Psychology of Women, and the International Stress Management Association. For more about Dr. King's courses and live challenges, visit her at EricaKKing.com.

Printed in the United States
By Bookmasters